Food Additive Toxicology

LIST OF FIGURES

LIST OF TABLES

LIST OF ABBREVIATIONS

6-GT	6-α-glucosyltransferase
ADI	acceptable daily intake
ALP	alkaline phosphatase
ALT	alanine aminotransferase
AST	aspartate aminotransferase
BHA	butylated □hydroxyanisole
BHT	butylated hydroxytoluene
BIRN	biomedical informatics research network
BPA	bisphenol-A
BST	bovine somatotropin
CAC	Codex Alimentarius Commission
CMC	carboxymethylcellulose
DDT	dichlorodiphenyltrichloroethane
DNA	deoxyribonucleic acid
EC	European Community
ECOTOX	ecotoxicology
EDI	estimated daily intake
EFSA	European Food Safety Authority
ERED	environmental residue-effects database
ES	electrophilic species
FAO	Food and Agricultural Organization
FDA	Food and Drug Administration
FSANZ	Food Standards Australia New Zealand
GIS	geographic information systems
GM	genetically modified
GRAS	generally recognized as safe
HCA	heterocyclic amines
HClO2	metastable chlorous acid

HFCS	high fructose corn syrup
HPD	household products database
HPLC	high-performance liquid chromatography
IARC	International Agency for the Research of Cancer
IAU	isoamylase activity units
ICH	International Conference on Harmonization
IMT	α-isomaltosyl transferase
JECFA	Joint FAO/WHO Expert Committee on Food Additives
LEU	Lecitase units
LO	level of concern
LOD	limit of detection
LOQ	limit of quantification
MSG	monosodium glutamate
NEPA	National Environmental Policy Act
NHANES	National Health and Nutrition Examination Survey
NLM	National Library of Medicine
NOAEL	no adverse effect level
NPA	network perturbation amplitude
PAH	polycyclic aromatic hydrocarbons
PCBs	polychlorinated biphenyls
PFOA	perfluorooctanoic acid
POPs	persistent organic pollutants
PVC	polyvinyl chloride
RPC	reversed phase chromatography
RP-HPLC	reversed-phase high-pressure liquid chromatography
TIP	toxicology information program
UV	ultraviolet
vCJD	variant creutzfeldt Jakob disease
WHO	World Health Organization

PREFACE

With the increasing amount of pollutants present in the environment, several other physical pollutants have been impacting the quality of food adversely. There are several unknown naturally occurring contaminants that find their way into food. The most ominous are products of mold growth called mycotoxins, which include carcinogenic aflatoxins. On the other hand, more than 2500 chemical substances are added to foods to modify or impart flavour, colour, stability, and texture, to fortify or enrich the nutritive value, or to reduce costs. In addition, an estimated 12,000 substances are used in such a way that they may unintentionally enter the food supply.

The book "Food Additive Toxicology" has been designed and structured in such a way that it would help the students gather knowledge about all those additives that are being used to adulterate the food and cause harm to human health. This book will help students understand that food additives are generally not consumed directly; rather, they are added to food intentionally to augment its processing or to improve aroma, colour, consistency, taste, texture, or shelf life. Additives are not considered "nutritional" even if they possess nutritive value.

The purpose of the book is to give an overview of certain risks that humans take while consuming food additives and certain problems that humans experience after consuming food additives. There is a plethora of information that opens a large field of applications to work on. This book intends to identify and come up with the best solution that is useful in dealing with those additives that are harmful to human health.

As it is defined in the book, "Toxicity classification is generally concerned with the classification of compounds based on their toxicity and their most important toxic effect. The compounds that have acute toxicity can be categorized into different categories such as allergenic, carcinogenic, neurotoxic, and several other compounds."

The information could be used to classify the compounds in such a structured way that a rating chart could be easily prepared to evaluate the compounds and measure the toxicity level. This will help in having a clear perception of food additives and their toxicity.

The subject of the book starts from providing a clear picture of several types of additives that are used in processed foods and about global regulations that have been framed against the usage of these harmful food additives.

The book further talks about the 12 most dangerous food additives and the ways that must be adopted to avoid using such additives. The most interesting part of the book comes when it talks about the differentiation between the artificial and natural flavour of additives that are used in food.

The next focus has been moved towards the clinical evaluation of the additives, where both qualitative and quantitative methods have been discussed descriptively. An attempt has been made to identify and estimate the synthetic food colours present in several food products.

Some sections would highlight technological innovation in the information resources in toxicology and the application of information resources in toxicology. This book will help to identify the core areas of additives and toxicology and their harmful impact on human health.

Chapter 1

Introduction to Food Toxicology

CONTENTS

Food toxicology is a discipline of science which is concerned with the evaluation and assessment of the toxic effects of certain substances present in food. In recent times, the complexity of food supply chain has increased. There have been alarming outbreaks of diseases which raised several issues involved in food safety. This chapter discusses food toxicity and food safety. It also details how food adulteration has existed since historical times. Toxin found in food is caused by various factors. This chapter lists down the various factors and describes in detail how they cause toxicity in food. There are various regulatory agencies that monitor food handling practices and the ingredients used by food processors. The chapter covers the role played by these agencies. Finally, the chapter explains what assessment of food toxicology means and the assessment of toxicity in humans.

1.1. INTRODUCTION

Food toxicology is a branch of science that is concerned with measuring and evaluating the harmful effects of certain chemicals present in the food, on the living beings that consumes it. These chemical agents can occur naturally or can be as a result of human factors. The former consists of plant toxins, microbes, and animal toxins. The latter comprises food additives, pesticides, contamination from the production process, or the packaging used.

Sometimes they are produced while preparing, processing, and preserving foods. These agents are mutagens and even carcinogenic. A study of food toxicology reveals the basic chemicals and the biological aspects of toxic substances are found in edible products.

The subject of food toxicology is now of high interest in the food industry, universities, and government agencies. Above all, it is the consumers who are now becoming more aware of food toxicology.

Toxicology has been defined as the study of the adverse effects of xenobiotics and thus is a borrowing science that has evolved from ancient poisoners. In the present day, toxicology is concerned beyond the study of the negative effects of exogenous agents to the study of molecular biology. It uses toxicants as tools.

In ancient times, toxicology was the foundation of therapeutics and medicine. In the present century, toxicology is fast growing subject. It continues to grow by absorbing information and methodologies from other branches of science like chemistry, biology, physics, and mathematics. This field now encompasses the safety evaluation and risk assessment.

Toxicologists work in a diverse field, and their activities are widespread. In the field of biomedical, they investigate the cause of serious and chronic illness caused as a result of exposure to chemicals. Toxicologists also work in the area of pharmacology and physiology by investigating physiological phenomena using toxic agents.

Toxicologists are involved in recognizing, quantifying, and identifying hazards resulting from occupational exposure to chemicals and the public health aspects of chemicals in the air, water, and other parts of the environment, foods, and drugs. In their conventional role's toxicologists have been closely associated with the invention and discovery of new medicines, pesticides, and drugs.

Another role of a toxicologist is in the development of standards and regulations that are established to safeguard humans and the ecosystem they live in from the negative effects of toxins. Another new subfield is environmental toxicology where the toxicologist is concerned with the effects of toxins on flora and fauna. Molecular toxicologists are studying the mechanisms by which toxicants modulate cell growth and differentiation, and cells respond to toxicants at the level of the gene.

All subfields of toxicology are concerned with studying the mechanism by which chemicals affect all ecosystems adversely. Clinical toxicology is concerned with finding a cure for the ill effects. It develops antidotes and other treatment methods to ameliorate poisonings and xenobiotic injury. They share methodologies for obtaining data about how poisonous, some materials can be. They then process the information carefully to predict the negative impact of the material on humans and their surroundings. There are various activities in this field that complement each other and form the field of toxicology.

1.2. FOOD TOXICITY AND SAFETY

It was largely believed that eating food in modern industrialized countries was considered a non-toxic activity. However, in recent times, many of the publicized alarming incidents concerning food safety made the consumer more aware about choosing food supply carefully. The food that humans consume is seldom subject to toxicological testing. Even then, their safety is not questioned.

It has been proved that all chemicals, even the ones that occur naturally in food, can be toxic beyond a certain limit. For instance, a high dose of salt and glucose can prove fatal in laboratory animals. Some vital nutrients like vitamin A and selenium can be toxic at doses, which are a few times higher than normal human requirements. There are some spices like pepper that have shown carcinogenic properties. Toxicity testing of a food or ingredient can tell us what the likely adverse effects are and at what level of consumption they may occur. However, this test alone does not reveal whether the food or ingredients can be consumed in normal quantities. The risk here is the possibility that the substance will be toxic under specific conditions of exposure (Figure 1.1).

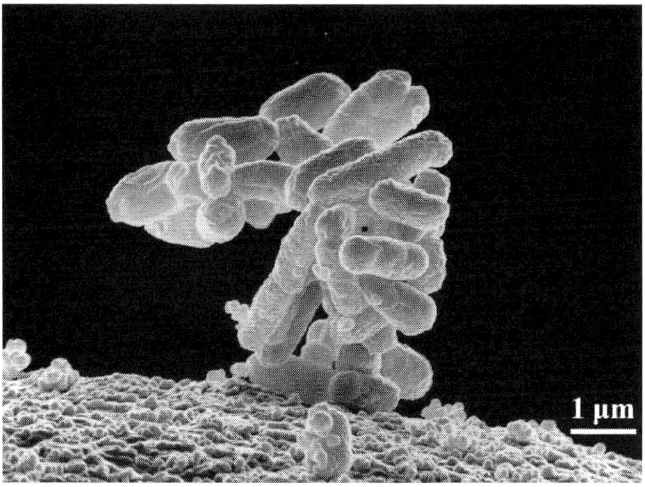

Figure 1.1. Representation of bacterial growth in small intestines.

Source: https://upload.wikimedia.org/wikipedia/commons/b/bc/E_coli_at_10000x%2C_original.jpg

The concept of risk considers various factors like the dosage of a particular chemical, the duration for which it is consumed, and the level of toxicity. It guides the safety of food. Toxicology is concerned not only with determining whether a food or ingredient is toxic or not. It attempts to establish whether consuming the food in normal amounts can increase the risk of illness.

Food adulteration has been a problem since historical times. In any urbanized society, most people eat food raised by others, and people depend on a chain of commerce that raises, transports, and sells food to consumers who are far from the countryside where most food originates. For instance, the US is inhibited by more than 300 million people, but less than one million people are a farmer. The rest of the population has to rely on these farmers and trust that the food is not toxic and has been grown according to law.

Only recently regulations were passed to control the production of food and their distribution. Before that, there were ample opportunities for adulteration. Adulteration results in the deterioration in the quality of food because of the addition of impure and inferior ingredients. This helped the unscrupulous food manufacturers and distributors to earn more profit. Food adulteration is a sad reality of urban society. The history of urban populations is intertwined with the history of food adulteration and the attempts to minimize it.

1.2.1. History of Food Adulteration

In the 18th and 19th centuries, European American cities were characterized by food adulteration. The increase in immigration increased the urban population. The food production could not remain localized anymore since it had to cater to the population situated in urban places. Consumers are now dependent entirely on intermediaries or middlemen for their supply of food.

The US witnessed the immigration from both rural areas and European cities, which increased its population. These urban people had little knowledge about how food was produced and handled, and the expected food quality. Food swindles were especially common among the large immigrant population of urban society as they often were the poorest and most powerless.

Frederich Accum published an expose, Adulteration of Food and Culinary Poison, and drew public attention to the toxic effects of food adulteration. He demonstrated how food adulteration was a reality. He came up with approaches to detect the presence of chemical additives and proved that they were common in the majority of the food. Metals were a common adulterant to add colour or modify the food. For instance, candies and pastries were often sold in bright colours to make them appealing. These colours were achieved by using copper or lead, both of which are toxic. They had a wide range of effects, including stomach upset, liver, and kidney damage, neurotoxicity, and in extreme cases, even death.

Similarly, copper washes were used to make green vegetables look fresher. Artificial tea was also introduced in the market. It made use of verdigris, which gave it the appearance of actual tea. The incidences of health issues and fatalities were increasing. Though the reasons are recognized now, back then the causes were unknown. By the 19th century, chemical additives were widely recognized as negative ingredients. Accum had managed to shape public opinion; however, he could not put an end to this practice.

Arthur Hill Hassall, a physician, also made a significant contribution to this field. He used a simple microscope for investigation purposes. The microscope revealed many non-chemical adulterants, which Accum was not able to detect because he used chemical analysis for his investigation. The adulterants consisted of plant leaves that were added to tea to increase their weight; alum was added to flour to improve its appearance etc. The results of these investigations eventually led to the enactment of laws to safeguard the consumers in England and the US.

Another group of contaminants is the organic pollutants which cause gastrointestinal infections and fatality. The supply chain now extends over long distances, which causes bacterial growth and spoilage of food. In the urban areas, the spoil for sold to factory workers after their long shifts who had no other alternative. The fresh foods would have been sold by then, and spoiled food was often camouflaged, not revealing its true state.

These revelations paved the way for passing legislation to secure food supply. Sinclair Lewis was a reformer of this period. He exposed that sausage was packed in the most unhygienic ways and included rats, their wastes, and even rat poison. President Roosevelt passes the Meat Inspection Act and the Pure Food and Drug Act in 1906 after an investigation revealed that Lewis's claims were true.

The nature and extent of food adulteration have changed over time. It is commonly believed that food is sufficiently clean and pure as we base our food handling techniques on sound knowledge of bacteriology. This assumption is far from true, and toxicities caused by food are still a growing threat. In recent times, the common causes of food recalls are a high level of metals like lead, bacterial contamination, and undeclared or mislabelled ingredients. The commonly avoided unhealthy foods like snacks and desserts do not contain any toxic contents that Accum had opposed. However, they have a very high sugar content, which makes them non-nutritious.

Food adulteration in the sense of ingredients added to increase profits has morphed subtly into food modification. In the present day, people do not consider preservatives as adulteration. Additives are omnipresent in the food; in some cases, they are adulterants and in some an improvement.

The additives are not only restricted to the preparation or distribution, and they are now used while growing as well. Pesticides and insecticides are commonly used to protect production from pests and improving yields. Besides, there are other contaminants that are accidental. Some common pollutants are persistent organic pollutants (POPs), pesticides, plasticizers, and metals. As conditions of growing and distributing food have changed, the question that Accum asked and answered in his day, still resonates, what exactly is really in our food?

1.3. TOXINS FOUND IN FOOD

Toxicities in foods occur mainly due to three causes:

- Microbial or environmental contamination;
- Naturally occurring toxins; and
- Addition of food additives.

The US Food and Drug Administration (FDA) classify the health hazards associated with food under the following categories. They have been ranked in descending order of seriousness.

- Microbiological contamination;
- Inappropriate eating habits;
- Environmental contamination;
- Natural toxic constituents;
- Pesticide residues;
- Food additives.

1.3.1. Microbial Contamination

- ***Pathogenic Bacteria*:** It causes acute gastroenteritis and can be caused by foodborne intoxication or foodborne infection. Staphylococcus aureus, Clostridium botulinum, Clostridium perfringens, and Salmonella species are the predominant pathogens and account for almost 80% of foodborne illnesses. Some causes of increasing foodborne illness are new types of pathogens, evolving food supply chain, and greater incidences of food being consumed away from home.
- ***Mycotoxin Mould*:** They generate a wide range of biologically active chemicals. They have been used to produce antibiotics. However, fungal products also contaminate food. Examples of such lethal compounds are Aflatoxins which are highly toxic and carcinogenic. They survive heat treatments and food processing. They are more common in tropical and semitropical parts of the world. Aflatoxin was discovered in peanuts first, and now maize is recognized as a major food containing this compound.

Patulin, an antibiotic derived from Penicillium claviforme, is carcinogenic as per a study on rats though not established. It is mostly found in rotten apples, and hence apple products may contain patulin. Fumonisins are carcinogenic mycotoxins from the Fusarium fungus associated with corn.

- ***New Foodborne Diseases:*** The most commonly known pathogens today, were unknown three decades ago. A new human pathogen known today is Campylobacter jejuni, which was earlier used in veterinary medicine. It occurs wherever raw meat is handled. Listeria monocytogenes is another common bacterium that is suppressed in freezing temperatures. It can lead to abortions and prove lethal in the case of the elderly, and those with low immunity. It occurs in milk, pâtés, soft cheese undercooked chicken, and frozen food.

Escherichia coli 0157:H7 damages the colon cells and causes bloody stools and pain in the abdomen. It mainly occurred in undercooked hamburger meat and causes outbreaks in the USA and Australia in the 90s. Another major pathogen in the 90s was Salmonella typhimurium, which caused outbreaks in the UK. It was multi-drug resistant, could survive low pH, and was hazardous in small numbers.

Norwalk virus is transferred from the feces of food handlers who do not maintain personal hygiene. Though it does not multiply, it remains active in food until it is consumed. 'Mad cow disease' (or BSE -bovine spongiform encephalopathy) is a slowly progressive and ultimately fatal neurological disorder of adult cattle that results from infection by a unique transmission agent called a prion. It first occurred in the UK in 1986 and later spread to Japan, Europe, and North America. Prion also causes the same infective variant Creutzfeldt Jakob Disease (vCJD), a disease affecting youth that may even cause death.

1.3.2. Environmental Contamination

Many environmental factors are responsible for food toxicities. They are discussed below:

- ***Heavy Metals and Minerals***: The most toxic element is Selenium. The levels in food are indicative of the levels in the soil. It occurs in high amounts in areas such as China and North Dakota. It causes gastrointestinal troubles and skin discolouration. In China in the early 1960s, selenium intoxication affected up to 50% of the population in certain villages, with brittle hair, skin lesions, and neurological disturbances the main symptoms.

- ***Mercury***: Fish contains high amounts of organic mercury, especially when their habitat contains a high level of mercury wastes. In the past, serious mercury poisoning had occurred in Japan and Iraq. In the latter, it occurred due to the bread made from wheat-containing traces of mercury-based pesticides.
- Cadmium is a toxic element that is found in biological systems. High levels of cadmium can cause chronic kidney failure. Cadmium levels in the soil increase due to phosphate fertilizers and pollutants. Plants absorb cadmium from the soil and are ingested by humans.
- ***Criminal Adulteration***: In the nineteenth century, there was an increased incidence of food adulteration to lower costs and increase profits. Milk is often contaminated with water, borax, vegetable oil, and detergents. In developed countries, high standards have been achieved by the food industry, thereby minimizing the risk of adulteration, but it is still a major problem in developing countries. Another adulterant found in cooking oil is aniline, which is used for industrial purposes. The Even baby formula is contaminated using Melamine to show high levels of protein.
- ***Packaging Materials***: The materials used for packing foods can also have toxic effects. Soldered metal cans are an example that was replaced by non-soldered ones. Bisphenol-A (BPA) is used in manufacturing synthetic resins and polycarbonate plastics. BPA is found in containers that come into contact with foodstuffs such as drinking vessels, baby bottles, and the internal coating on cans for tinned food. It mimics certain hormones and harms the reproductive system. It also harms the development of infants and young children. Hence BPA free bottles were introduced for; however, it is still being used in the manufacture of bottles and containers used for storing consumables.
- ***Industrial Pollution***: The industrial era has been characterized by many hazardous pollutants being emitted into the atmosphere and their subsequent infusion into the food chain. Polychlorinated biphenyls (PCBs) are a major hazard that is used in various products

like paints, lubricants, and plastics. Although manufacture has now ceased, their stability and lipid solubility has meant that they accumulate in fatty tissue and they have become widespread, particularly in seafood. The extent of their prevalence is so high that it can be found in traces in human milk. They are perceived to be mild carcinogens and can cause development problems in children and fetuses.

- ***Radioactive Fallout*:** The most important dangerous radioisotopes in fall-out are strontium-90 and cesium-137, with half-lives of 28 and 30 years. Strontium is absorbed by the body and stored in bones. It is found in high levels in milk and hence dangerous for children and infants. In 1963, post the Nuclear Test Ban Treaty, the level of radioactive pollutants has decreased remarkably. However, instances of accidental exposure have been noted, which leads to food poisoning.
- ***Changes During Cooking or Processing*:** Exposure to high heat during cooking can cause the carbonization of food and make it carcinogenic. The major compounds are polycyclic aromatic hydrocarbons (PAH), produced mainly by the burning of fats, and heterocyclic amines (HCA) produced from amino acids. Barbequing of food can also lead to carcinogenic formation. Acrylamide also occurs in food rich in starch when it is cooked at a high temperature. Although the exact effects of acrylamide are not yet determined, all food regulatory authorities encourage the adoption of cooking methods that will minimize its formation in foods.

Irradiation is used to sterilize foods and increase their shelf life; however, it has been met with resistance from consumer groups since it may release potentially toxic chemicals. Researchers concluded that there was a harmful effect of irradiation and is approved by WHO as a safe process.

1.3.3. Natural Toxins

Toxic compounds occur naturally in many plants and animals. Unlike man-made toxic compounds like pesticides, drugs, emissions, additives they are inherent to the food. When consumed beyond permissible limits, they have serious implications, including fatality. It may be serving a particular function or may have evolved as a defence mechanism. Various types of chemicals are found in nature which varies in nature and toxicity.

- ***Natural Toxins Present in Food of Plant Origin*:** There are over 2,000 plant species in the world that have natural toxins present in them. Wild berries, mushrooms often cause poisoning. Only a hundred species of plants are recognized as edible worldwide. Some of these plants can also become toxic if they are consumed in excess or not treated well. Depending on the species, the edible parts of plants vary, which may include foliage, buds, stems, roots, fruits, and tubers, and so are their poisonous parts.

  Plants belonging to the same species may not necessarily exhibit the same levels of toxicities. It is also dependent on the geographical conditions of its habitat. Plant organs that are the key to survival and reproduction will have these compounds at elevated levels. These compounds may for at a faster rate in some critical stages, for instance in buds, seedlings, or young tissues. Glycoalkaloid is a natural toxin found in potatoes. Cyanide generating compounds are found in bamboo shoots and apricot seeds. Lectins and enzyme inhibitors are present in soya beans, legumes, and green beans.

- ***Natural Toxins Present in Food of Animal Origin*:** Natural toxins occur in animals as a result of metabolism or a chemical that it ingests. Although terrestrial animals causing food poisoning are uncommon, marine toxins are common. Microalgae are toxic creatures that release marine toxins. These are accumulated in finfish, shellfish, and crustaceans which are passed on to humans. Tetrodotoxin is a potent neurotoxin that is produced by certain bacteria. Pufferfish is a major carrier of tetrodotoxin, and even a small dose causes a fatality.

Ciguatoxin, which is found in over 300 species of fish, causes seafood poisoning. Histamine is released when scombroid fish is spoiled by bacterial contamination cause seafood poisoning.

Almost 1,200 species of animals have been recognized as poisonous to date. Though the majority of them are not consumed, the ones that are should be thoroughly treated before consumption. Glands of some animals that are not considered poisonous or venomous when ingested can also cause food poisoning such as the gallbladder of grass carp, which contains cyprinol related chemicals (Figure 1.2).

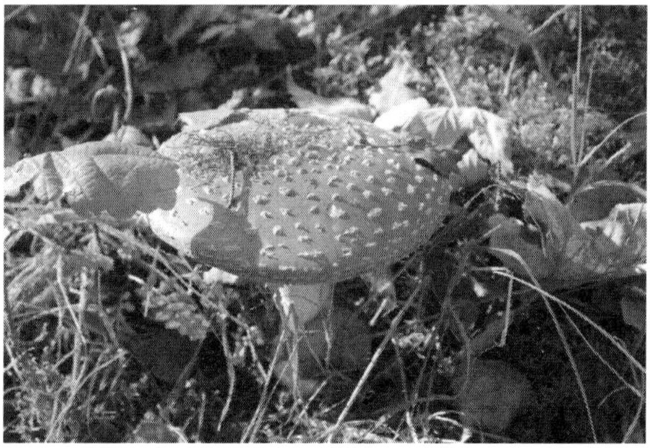

Figure 1.2. Certain mushrooms have toxic effects on humans.

Source: https://pxhere.com/en/photo/348042

- ***Toxic Effects and Food Poisoning*:** Natural toxins in food when ingested can cause various symptoms and lead to both acute and chronic health effects. Some of the acute symptoms are neurological symptoms, mild gastrointestinal upset, respiratory paralysis to fatality. Children and the elderly are vulnerable to these symptoms. The effects of acute symptoms can be noticed immediately after consumption of toxic seafood. Ingestion of wild mushrooms or improperly treated apricot and ginkgo also causes acute poisoning.

Chronic toxicity is caused by alkaloids, which are present in plants. Pyrrolizidine alkaloids are found in weeds in crops and some other plants which can damage the liver when consumed for long periods. The toxic effects and the symptoms depend on the level of toxins present as well as the vulnerability of each individual.

- ***Risk Reduction Measures*:** Certain toxins can be eliminated or reduced by using appropriate methods of food processing. In cases where it is not possible to effectively treat the food, they should be avoided. Enzyme inhibitors and lectins can be destroyed by thorough cooking. Certain cyanide-producing compounds can be eliminated by soaking them in water and boiling them. In some fishes, only certain parts are toxic like the skin, gonads, and removing them eliminates toxins present in their tissues.

In general, whether a substance poses harm depends on its concentration, amount of intake, and the health status of the individual since the body can detoxify low levels of many potentially dangerous substances. The adoption is established ways of processing food that is known to remove toxins that can reduce the risk of food poisoning. Besides, it is important to maintain a balanced and varied diet, so the intake of certain natural toxins can be contained to an acceptable level.

1.3.4. Agricultural Residues

- ***Pesticides*:** Farmers use pesticides to protect crops from pests, microbes, and insects. Pesticides have toxic effects, both acute and chronic, on humans. The symptoms depend on the quantity and how an individual is exposed to these chemicals. In earlier days, the pesticides used remained in soil and water for years. While the developed countries have banned them, many developing countries still use them. The farmers are exposed to pesticides the most and hence, face the highest health risk.

Pesticides are important for modern-day cultivation. They increase yields by preserving them and increasing the number of times crops can be cultivated on the same land. This helps in achieving food security in developing countries. WHO has taken steps to reduce the harmful effects of pesticides? It reviews evidence and establishes the permissible threshold for the residues. Currently, over 1000 types of pesticides are being used around the world to protect crops. The properties and impact of this pesticide vary.

Dichlorodiphenyltrichloroethane (DDT) and lindane are some pesticides that can be found in the water and soil even years after its use. These chemicals have been banned by countries that signed the 2001 Stockholm Convention – an international treaty that aims to eliminate or restrict the production and use of POPs.

Some pesticides are more harmful than others. For instance, insecticides are more toxic than herbicides. Similarly, the amount of pesticide used also has determined the effects on the people exposed to it. Another factor is the susceptibility of each individual to these toxins. Finally, the route of exposure also determines the nature and level of impact. The various routes include inhaling, ingesting, skin contact, etc.

Foods that allow for international trade cannot contain pesticides that are genotoxic, i.e., damage the genes or cause cancer. People who are exposed to prolonged exposure to pesticides in large quantities can have acute poisoning, and other adverse impact on health like issues is reproduction and cancer.

Pesticides are one of the primary causes of death in developing countries. Since pesticides are inherently toxic and intentionally used in the environment. Hence the production and use of pesticides and should be strictly monitored. It is also important to regulate the residue in food and the environment.

The people who are directly exposed to pesticides, like the agricultural workers and other people inhabiting the area where pesticides are used. The other people who are far away from the areas where pesticides are used are exposed to residues through water and food, which are much lower than direct exposure.

- ***Hormones*:** These are chemical substances that convey specific signals in the regulation of endogenous processes within the body. Hormones naturally occur in muscle meat, kidneys, and liver, which enable endogenous processes. Some hormones like testosterone, progesterone, and estrogen occur in higher levels in milk compared to muscle meat or other organs which are consumed, eggs, fish, and vegetables.

The majority of the intake of these hormones in humans comes from milk. Both naturally occurring hormones and artificial ones are similar in the way they affect the mechanism at the receptor. However, some synthetic ones can take a longer time to metabolize and hence be retained in the body longer.

The European Union does not permit the use of hormones. Hormones were used to fatten cattle to improve the animal feed conversion ratio. It carried significant health risks and hence was banned in the EU in 1988. Hormones can also be used in livestock farming for breeding and therapeutic purposes. In Germany, the regional authority controls the use -of pharmacologically effective substances. They regularly inspect food to detect the use of unauthorized hormones.

Bovine somatotrophin (BST) is used to improve the yields of milk and meat. Many countries find the use of BST objectionable. Although low levels of BST can be detected in the milk of treated cows, the hormones are inactive in humans and are digested and inactivated in the stomach when consumed in food. In 1993, it was approved by the FDA since the effects on a human were considered negligible; however, it is not used in many countries on animal welfare grounds.

Milk for human consumption is acquired from animals that contain hormones. Progesterone and estrogens are naturally occurring hormones.

However, consumption in normal quantities results in very low ingestion compared to the natural self-synthesis of these hormones in humans. Moreover, they get metabolized quickly. Currently, the risks associated with hormone ingestion milk intake are low.

1.3.5. Food Additives

Food additives have been used for ages to make the food look more appealing, enhance its flavour, and preserve it for a longer time. In the current lifestyle, the urban population spends a significant portion of their budget on processed food, which exposes them to many artificial food additives and the subsequent health effect. Some of the additives are discussed below.

- ***Artificial Sweeteners*:** Aspartame is found in food that is labeled sugar-free or diet food. This additive is believed to be carcinogenic and has a profound health impact. It also affects short-term memory and intelligence, chronic fatigue, depression, headaches, dizziness, migraines, and seizures. Other significant risks include lymphoma, brain tumour, multiple sclerosis, diabetes, Alzheimer's, Parkinson's, and fibromyalgia.

A relatively new artificial sweetener, Acesulfame-K, is used in baking goods, gum, and gelatin. Though its effects are not fully known, it has been linked to a kidney tumor. These sweeteners are found in diet sodas, jelly, desserts, ice tea, toothpaste, etc.

- ***High Fructose Corn Syrup (HFCS):*** It is a very popular syrup that contains highly refined sugar. It is used in the majority of the processed food. It causes obesity, raises LDL, diabetes, and tissue damage besides other toxic effects. It is used in foods like bread, flavoured yogurt, canned vegetables, salad dressings, and cereals.
- ***Monosodium Glutamate (MSG/E621):*** MSG is a flavour enhancer used in noodles, chips, soups, frozen food, and many dishes made in restaurants. It is an amino acid and a known excitotoxin. It can overexcite the cells and may even result in death. Regular intake of MSG includes eye damage, depression, headaches, disorientation, and obesity. It encourages overeating and subsequent obesity. It is widely used in Chine foods as a seasoning.
- ***Trans-Fat:*** Trans-fat is used as a preservative and recognized as one of the most toxic additives. It is formed by a process called hydrogenation and is found in certain processed food and deep-

fried food which contain margarine or partially hydrogenated vegetable oils. It is the cause of many health problems like heart attacks, strokes, diabetes, inflammation, an increase in LDL, and a decrease in HDL. It is found in baked goods, chips, crackers, fast food, and margarine (Figure 1.3).

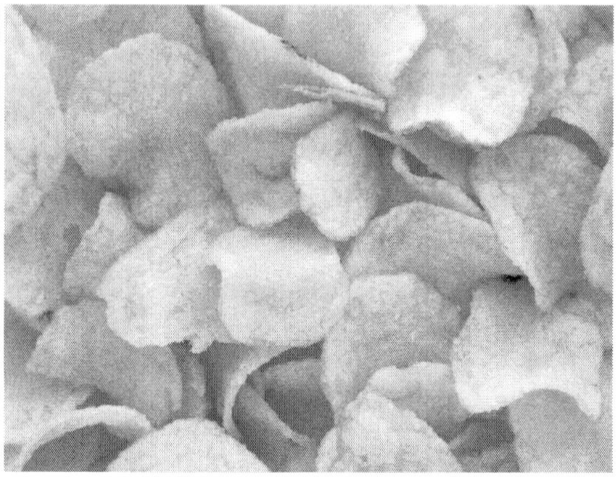

Figure 1.3. Potato chips contain trans fats and artificial flavours.

Source: https://upload.wikimedia.org/wikipedia/commons/6/69/Potato-Chips.jpg

- ***Common Food Dyes:*** Artificial colours or food dyes because behavioural issues in children, affects cognitive ability. Food colouring has been known to cause cancer in animals. E133 which imparts a blue colour to food is banned in Finland, Norway, and France as it may lead to chromosomal damage. It is used in candy, pet food, cakes, soft drinks, etc.

E124 is a red dye that is used in maraschino cherries, fruit cocktails, candy, bakery products, ice creams, and more. It is linked with thyroid cancer and chromosomal damage. E110 and E102 are used in yellow-coloured foods. It is found in candy, soft drinks, cheese, and macaroni. It can lead to the adrenal gland and kidney tumor.

- ***Sodium Sulfite:*** It is a preservative that is found in wine and other processed foods. As per the FDA 1% of the population, the majority of who are asthmatic are sensitive to sulfites in food. Such people experience breathing problems, headaches, and rashes. In some serious cases, it may even lead to cardiac arrest.
- ***Sodium Nitrate/Sodium Nitrite:*** Sodium nitrate is a colouring,

flavouring agent, and preservative. It is found in ham, corned beef, smoked fish, processed meat, and hot dogs. It is highly carcinogenic as well. Inside the human digestive system, it forms a variety of nitrosamine compounds that enter the bloodstream and wreak havoc with some internal organs: the liver and pancreas in particular.

Although USDA tried to ban this additive in the 1970s, the food manufacturers did not let this happen, and it is still widely used since it keeps meat bright red in colour. Hence stale meat looks fresh and vibrant. Hotdogs, lunch meat, corned beef, bacon, ham, cured meats, smoked fish, or any other type of processed meat are sources of sodium nitrate.

- ***BHA and BHT (E320):*** Butylated hydroxyanisole (BHA) and butylated hydroxytoluene (BHT) are used by manufacturers of cereals, potato chips, chewing gum, and vegetable oils. It is a preservative that retains the food colour, flavour, and prevents the food from becoming rancid. It can also form cancer-causing compounds in the human body. It is found in gum, cereal, potato chips, lard, frozen sausage, candy jelly.
- ***Sulfur Dioxide (E220):*** It is found in soft drinks, juices, wine, dried fruits, and potato products. The FDA has banned its use in raw fruit and vegetables. It causes bronchial problems, hypotension, flushing, and anaphylactic shock. It is prohibited for people suffering from asthma, cardiovascular diseases, conjunctivitis, and emphysema.

1.3.6. Novel Foods

Technological advancement has led to the invention of many new food ingredients and foods that were not used earlier. Many of them have been developed to improve nutrition. Some of the novel foods include genetically modified (GM) foods, new algal sources of Omega 18, artificial fat substitutes, and phytosterols.

It is a complex task to assess whether GM foods will have any long-term impacts. The assessment would require feeding high doses of the foods which would make their diets nutritionally unbalanced.

Moreover, animals may refuse to eat when they are offered the same foods in large quantities. These difficulties and welfare concerns about the use of animal studies that were unlikely to result in meaningful information led to the development of the concept of 'substantial equivalence,' particularly

food us silver, zinc, and titanium oxide. They are mainly used in nutritional supplements and food packing. However, studies reveal that size alone is not a factor for determining safety. Risk assessment is required for the novelty and not size alone.

1.4. REGULATORY AGENCIES

All regulators use similar techniques to evaluate scientific evidence and measure food safety. However, various countries adopt different management styles for food safety legislation. In 1963, the Food and Agricultural Organization (FAO) and the World Health Organization (WHO) established the Codex Alimentarius Commission (CAC) (Codex).

The purpose was to develop international guidelines, standards, and codes of practice to address the issues in food composition and safety and making food regulations across countries (Figure 1.4).

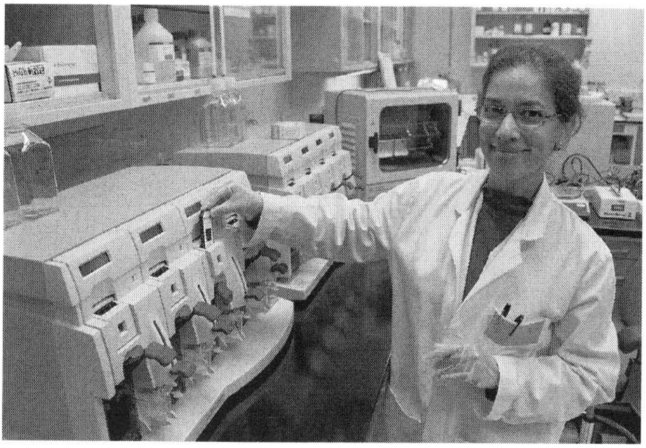

Figure 1.4. Representation of Toxicology Research Center in FDA.

Source: https://upload.wikimedia.org/wikipedia/commons/thumb/b/be/Toxicology_Research_at_FDA_%28NCTR_1179%29_%286008495329%29.jpg/800px-Toxicology_Research_at_FDA_%28NCTR_1179%29_%286008495329%29.jpg

At present Codex have over 165 members. Though Codex standards are not binding on individual countries, they have a considerable influence and are the basis of yardstick for World Trade Organization agreements. Some examples are Technical Barriers to trade and the Application of Sanitary and Phytosanitary Measures. They compel the countries to establish food standards that are in line with the Codex. In the US, the FDA develops standards for food composition, quality, and safety as well as being responsible for approval of therapeutic drugs and cosmetics. It also discharges the responsibility of food inspection and food monitoring. The FDA is a respected authority globally. It works like the GRA listing is of the highest quality because of resourcing of expert scientific staff.

In Australia, Foods Standards Australia New Zealand, which is a bi-national authority, is responsible for setting standards for manufactured foods in these two countries. This includes standards for additives and contaminants. It also checks for the safety of novel foods. Primary food production and foodservice safety standards are set separately in each country. In Australia, the State Governments are responsible for ensuring compliance and the national agency, which sets these standards.

In Britain, the Foods Standards Agency acts as an autonomous body for ensuring food safety. It was established in 2000 to safeguard the consumer interest and public health raised by the BSE outbreaks. The FSA acts as an advisor to the Government and public on food safety measures that can be adopted when food travels from farm to fork. It safeguards the consumer interest by enforcing regulations and monitoring the food practices adopted by the manufacturers.

In 2002, the European Food Safety Authority (EFSA) was established in Europe to provide scientific advice as an independent body concerning matters of food and feed safety. EFSA principally deals with requests for risk assessments from the European Commission, Parliament, and Council and plans to take on a wider brief from other European institutions shortly.

The primary responsibility of all regulatory agencies is assessing risks related to food security and managing them. Risk assessment is a scientific step that involves the following steps:

- Identifying the biological, physical, and chemical agents that are potential hazards and may harm the human body.
- Quantitative and qualitative assessment of hazards, including the effects of various doses. This is called hazard characterization.
- Assessing the exposure risk that is the risk of ingestion of toxins from food considering the typical dietary patterns.
- Forecasting the probability and the extent of the negative impact, which is called risk characterization.

Risk management is the process of weighing policy options in the light of the risk assessment results and selecting appropriate control measures. Control can be exercised by restricting certain ingredients in food completely. This includes some carcinogenic ingredients. Another control option includes setting the threshold level for certain foods like agricultural residues and additives. Good manufacturing practices have to be established and monitored.

Labeling requirements should be laid down for warning consumers about potential allergens. Most importantly, public awareness should be raised through public education about safe and hazardous food. Risk communication is the process of making the risk management information comprehensible to food producers, policymakers, and consumers.

1.5. ASSESSMENT OF FOOD TOXICOLOGY

The history of food toxicity can be traced back to the era of Hippocrates when he made a statement that "Let food be thy medicine and medicine thy food." This statement was made over two millennia ago. There has been a significant advancement in the field of food toxicology with the development of biochemistry, cell culture techniques, molecular biology. It is now easier to identify and classify ingredients that could be toxic.

Mechanistic insights obtained by evaluating toxicity in food by employing various models have helped improve food safety. These models include in vitro biochemical, in vitro to clinical settings, cell-based in vitro.

Two connected aspects of measuring the presence of toxicants in the food are:

- Actual measurement of the effects of toxicants in different models ranging from in vitro biochemical systems, cell-based in vitro systems, animal in vivo models to clinical settings analyzing systemic or organ-specific toxicity; and
- Evaluation of ingredients or substances present in food that could be a potential toxicant.

These two areas are linked because the mechanistic knowledge obtained by evaluating the actual impact of toxicants can lead to the identification of other possible toxicants in food. The field of pharmacology has contributed the maximum to the evaluation of food toxicology. The field of nutritional science and pharmacology has a common origin. Many of the common drugs that are used in the world have been obtained from natural products.

The impact of many toxicants converges on the generation of electrophilic species (ES). This results in chronic inflammation and oxidative stress. Toxicants can cause oxidative reactions, which will result in a buildup of damaged macromolecules, which could impair cells, tissue, and organs. Therefore, toxicants can cause cell deaths, aging, chronic inflammations, and degenerative diseases like Parkinson's, Alzheimer's, and Huntington's diseases. There are other diseases like myocardial infarction, multiple sclerosis, arteriosclerosis, rheumatoid arthritis, cataracts, diabetes, sterility, and others.

In vitro assessment is facilitated by various biochemical systems which aid in analyzing the destructive effects on the activity and integrity of key biomolecules. Such molecules are significant to maintain metabolism, integrity, signaling pathways besides gene expression and translation. On a cellular level, a variety of viability assays are routinely used to quantify the effects of potential food toxicants for extrapolation of the range of dosages used for maximally tolerated concentrations for in vivo animal models and also clinical settings.

Mechanistic insights were gathered from the development of many cell-based in vitro systems. These were developed by amalgamating with targeted in vitro analysis. These analyses concentrated on receptor-dependent pathways and specific key enzymes. Although in vivo rodent models are perhaps the most effective assessment models. However, it has certain drawbacks like high costs, ethical issues, inconsistent reports, low throughput readouts, and concerns of extrapolability to humans.

New strategies have emerged, and the paradigm in toxicology has switched from the traditional apical endpoint approach as determined in animal models to a mechanism-based approach by in silico methods. Biomarkers that are specific to a cell on protein, gene, or metabolite levels can be measured using toxicoproteomics, toxicogenomics, or toxicometabonomics. Food toxicology data that are derived from in vitro biochemical, in vivo animal, and silico systems have contributed mechanistic knowledge about toxicity in humans. It also enabled the use of surrogate biomarkers in clinical settings.

The introduction of alternative surrogate animals belonging to the lower hierarchy has advanced the toxicity assessment. Some model installation includes fruit flies, zebrafish, or nematodes. These models are considered better than the traditional rodent models. This is because they are considered more ethical and have high throughput. These sub-mammalian vertebrate and invertebrate models are considered effective. This is because there is a great homology of genes between humans and the nematodes, zebrafish, and fruit flies. Food toxicology has advanced significantly, which has made the drug and food safety prediction rate more accurately. These dimensions were behind comprehension a decade back.

1.5.1. Toxicity Assessment in Humans

There are various areas of toxicology involved in assessing toxicity caused by food in humans. This comprises forensic, environmental, and regulatory toxicology. Evaluation of body fluids and biopsy of tissues can help in assessing the toxicants present in humans. Clinical toxicology is mainly based on analyzing genotoxicity, neurotoxicity, cardiotoxicity, hepatotoxicity, nephrotoxicity, carcinogenicity, immunotoxicity, food allergy, and/or endocrine disruption as they affect a variety of disorders.

Much of the information about toxicity in humans has been gathered by conducting a post mortem analysis of the molecules and atoms of cells, tissues, and organs. Forensic toxicology is also closely associated with toxicological pathology. However, it deals with satisfying legal requirements. Environmental toxicology is concerned with assessing various biological, chemical, and physical agents which are toxic for humans. Regulatory toxicology is related to the risk assessment of food and potential toxicants.

There have been considerable advancements in the field of nanotechnology and is now applied in the food industry. This gave rise to the new discipline of nanotoxicology, which studies the potential risks and the safety of nanoparticles.

Some studies point out that GM organisms and food can also be toxic. The different sub-fields concerned with toxicity in humans are not independent by intertwining. The objective of all these subfields is to gain knowledge about the toxicants that are hazardous so that their intake can be prevented, and food safety can be ensured.

Surrogate biomarker molecules are quite useful in clinical toxicology, and they indicate the extent of tissue and organ damage. The major advancement in the field of biotechnology has made these biomarker predictions more accurate since their specificity and sensitivity levels have drastically improved. The biomarkers that help in identifying negative biological impact can be classified into two types:

- Biomarkers assessing function and integrity of cells and tissues which are typically tissue-specific cytoplasmic enzymes that leak from damaged or dying cells and can be monitored in blood or urine; and

- Biomarkers indicate the damage caused to cells and tissues based on the responses of inducible defence systems.

The data generated by the mentioned approaches are considered as the first step of toxicity assessment. Histology is used to validate this assessment, and this may lead to causative relationships relevant to degenerative diseases.

1.6. CONCLUSION

In the present day, there are various potential health risks associated with food. The increase in urbanization had made localized production of food not feasible. Food is transported long distances from rural to urban areas. Many toxins occur naturally or due to natural processes. Moreover, with the advancement in technology, new additives, preservatives, and enhancers have been invented, which has many toxic effects.

One of the significant sources of food toxicities is biological agents like disease-causing bacteria, fungi, bacteria, and certain seafood. Factors like mass production of food, longer food supply chains; increased incidence of eating out have led to the generation of new pathogens. This implies that foodborne illness will remain the primary cause of food toxicities.

JECFA assesses the safety of food additives at a global level. At the national level, each country is responsible for establishing its regulations and standards. GM foods, novel foods, and nano-materials pose new challenges for traditional safety assessment processes, but as the food supply becomes increasingly global, food regulations about food safety are becoming more harmonized internationally. Radioactive elements, some metals, and packaging materials that are used by food processors also cause toxicities in food.

Food toxicology is concerned with the study of the characteristics, nature, detection, and implication of toxic ingredients in food and how they cause diseases in humans. It mainly deals with ensuring food safety. Some important considerations in the field of toxicology are natural food components, food adulterants, and additives. The increased use of these ingredients has made it an urgent need to devise new high-throughput testing approaches which will help assess the toxicity present in foods that poses a significant health hazard. Currently, toxicology is observing a patterned shift in the evaluation of chemical hazards in food safety.

REFERENCES

1. Assessing, Managing, and Communicating Chemical Food Risks – IFT.org (2017). [online] Ift.org. Available at: http://www.ift.org/knowledge-center/read-ift-publications/science-reports/scientific-status-summaries/assessing-managing-and-communicating-chemical-food-risks.aspx (Accessed on 14 May 2019).
2. FST 128 – Food Toxicology | Food Science and Technology. (2019). [online] Foodscience.ucdavis.edu. Available at: https://foodscience.ucdavis.edu/academic-programs/undergraduate/courses/fst-128-food-toxicology (Accessed on 14 May 2019).
3. Pesticide Residues in Food. (2018). [online] Who.int. Available at: https://www.who.int/news-room/fact-sheets/detail/pesticide-residues-in-food (Accessed on 14 May 2019).
4. Questions and Answers on Hormones in Meat and Milk – BfR. (2014). [online] Bfr.bund.de. Available at: https://www.bfr.bund.de/en/questions_and_answers_on_hormones_in_meat_and_milk-191516.html (Accessed on 14 May 2019).
5. Gallo, M., (2019). History and Scope of Toxicology | Casarett and Doull's Toxicology: The Basic Science of Poisons, 8e | AccessPharmacy | McGraw-Hill Medical. [online] Accesspharmacy.mhmedical.com. Available at: https://accesspharmacy.mhmedical.com/content.aspx?bookid=958&sectionid=53483720 (Accessed on 14 May 2019).
6. Mercola, J., (2010). Top 10 Food Additives to Avoid. [online] Foodmatters.com. Available at: https://www.foodmatters.com/article/top-10-food-additives-to-avoid (Accessed on 14 May 2019).
7. Schell, M. L., Schell, M., & Cook, K., (2012). What's NOT to Eat- Food Adulteration in the Context of Human Biology. [online] NCBI. Available at: https://www.ncbi.nlm.nih.gov/pmc/articles/PMC3275668/ (Accessed on 14 May 2019).
8. Tang, S. P. D., (2019). An Overview of Natural Toxins in Food. [online] Cfs.gov.hk. Available at: https://www.cfs.gov.hk/english/multimedia/multimedia_pub/multimedia_pub_fsf_11_02.html (Accessed on 14 May 2019).
9. Williams, P., (2012). Food Toxicity and Safety. [online] Pdfs.semanticscholar.org. Available at: https://pdfs.semanticscholar.org/5929/c425e7253093792dc9751fd9616c996507b7.pdf (Accessed on 14 May 2019).

Chapter 2

Science and Principles of Toxicology

CONTENTS

The toxicology is the study of the toxic effects of the chemical compounds or food additives that create several toxic syndromes in living organisms. There are several important concepts and principles that play an important role in understanding several concepts in toxicology of living organisms. The important concepts relating the toxicology of living organisms such as the toxicity, xenobiotics, hazard, risk, toxicity rating and toxicity classification, absorption, gastrointestinal absorption, elimination have been explained in details. There are three basic principles related to the toxic responses that are generated in living organisms and these three principles have been explained in detail. The principles related to the food additives in toxicology and the safety evaluation in toxicology have been explained in detail. There is need to understand these several principles in toxicology to understand the impact of the food additives on the living organisms and the different types of food additives that are allowed or not allowed in several organisms.

2.1. INTRODUCTION TO IMPORTANT CONCEPTS OF TOXICOLOGY

2.1.1. Toxicity

Toxicity refers to the internal capacity of any chemical agent to affect the organism adversely.

2.1.2. Xenobiotics

Xenobiotics are a concept that refers to "foreign substances," which indicates few organisms that are foreign to the organisms. Xenobiotics are those substances that include several drugs, industrial chemicals, naturally occurring poisons, and several other environmental pollutants.

2.1.3. Hazard

Hazard is a concept that refers to those organisms that have the potential for toxicity in a particular situation or setting.

2.1.4. Risk

Risk refers to the probability of a particular adverse effect to happen. Risk is a term that is generally expressed as the percentage of cases that have come up from a particular population during a specific period. A risk estimate is a variable that is generally derived based upon the actual cases that are present or the projection of future cases that is obtained based on the extrapolations.

2.1.5. Toxicity Rating and Toxicity Classification

The rating of toxicity of several compounds and the classification of toxicity of certain compounds is known to be extremely important in the regulatory purposes of certain compounds.

2.1.6. Toxicity Rating

Toxicity rating refers to the random classification of compounds based on the toxicity and exposure levels of certain compounds. The toxicity grading can be used to label or categorize compounds into several categories such as "super-toxic," "highly toxic," "moderately toxic," and several others in a similar manner. The most common methods of toxicity rating are mostly concerned with acute toxicity of the compounds.

Toxicity classification is generally concerned with the classification of compounds based on their toxicity and their most important toxic effect. The compounds that have acute toxicity can be categorized into different categories, such as allergenic, carcinogenic, neurotoxic, and several other compounds. The toxicity rating and classification of compounds would play an important role in giving a warning or information regarding these compounds.

2.1.7. Dose-Effect Relationship

The dose-effect relationship is used to explain the effect that is caused in human beings on the consumption of a certain dose of compounds. An increase in the concentration of the dose or exposure to the chemical may increase the effect of the result or may lead to severe consequences in human beings.

The dose-effect relationship may be used to draw a curve that is used to determine the dose-response relationship of the chemical. There could be a dose-effect curve that can be drawn at the level of an organism, cell, or an entire target molecule. Some severe toxic effects are generated as a response to certain toxic effects, and these may be as severe as death or cancer. These effects are generally called "all or none" effects.

The dose-response relationship is a relationship that is present between the dose of a chemical compound that is exposed to human beings and the percentage of the exposed individuals who are showing a specific effect. The increase in the dose of a compound would lead to a larger number of people who are exposed to a particular drug being affected by the toxic effects.

The dose-effect and dose-response relationships in toxicology are known to be extremely important concepts in toxicology. Different types of dose-response curves can be obtained for a particular chemical. A majority of the dose-response curves for several toxic effects are known to be in sigmoid shape.

- **Latency Time:** It is known to be the time between the initial exposure to the chemical and the appearance of a specific effect or response of a particular chemical. The latency time is generally the time that is used for the generation of several carcinogenic effects in human beings.
- **LD_{50} (effective dose):** It is known to be that particular dose that is known to cause nearly 50% lethality in the entire animal population.
- **NOEL:** It refers to the no observed adverse effect level in human beings and the highest dose that is known to cause several toxic effects in human beings. Establishing a NOEL requires multiple doses, a large population, and additional information to make sure that the absence of a response is not merely a statistical phenomenon.
- **LOEL:** It is the lowest observed effective dose on a dose-response curve or the lowest dose that causes an effect.

2.1.8. Absorption

Absorption refers to the uptake of a chemical from the environment into the organism. Absorption is a term that generally refers to the entry of the chemical substance into the human body by crossing the barrier tissues and entering into the circulatory system. The chemicals that enter the circulatory system are transported to several parts of the body through the circulatory system. The absorption of a chemical or a food additive generally happens through several routes of exposure. There are several routes for absorption and different types of absorption are as follows:

- Pulmonary absorption;
- Percutaneous absorption;
- Gastrointestinal absorption;
- Other routes of absorption.

1. ***Pulmonary Absorption:*** Pulmonary absorption is the mode of absorption where chemicals are absorbed into the body through the lungs. This generally happens because of the absorption of the chemicals by inhalation of these chemicals. The inhalation of toxic chemicals is the most hazardous way to generate adverse effects in the human body.

   Pulmonary absorption is the most hazardous route of absorption because it is the quickest channel for a hazardous chemical to enter into the circulatory system of the human body and generate adverse effects in their system.

2. ***Percutaneous Absorption*:** Percutaneous absorption generally refers to the route of absorption where the chemicals are absorbed into the human body because of the absorption through the skin of human beings. Skin is known to be an effective barrier in human beings that protects human beings from any potential harmful effects. Skin is known to maintain thermoregulatory balance in human beings, protect human beings from micro-organisms, ultraviolet (UV) radiations, deleterious agents, and excessive loss of water.

Though the skin is an effective barrier, several chemicals can be absorbed by the skin and enter into the circulatory system. Several fat-soluble compounds are absorbed by the skin into the circulatory system, and they are known to get quickly absorbed into the system. Percutaneous absorption of vapor may be important for solvents with very low vapor pressure and high affinity to water and skin.

2.1.9. Gastrointestinal Absorption

Gastrointestinal absorption is known to be a route of absorption where the food is ingested into the system because of the absorption of chemicals. This is a process of ingestion that generally happens because of the consumption of any food which can initiate a toxic response in human beings (Figure 2.1).

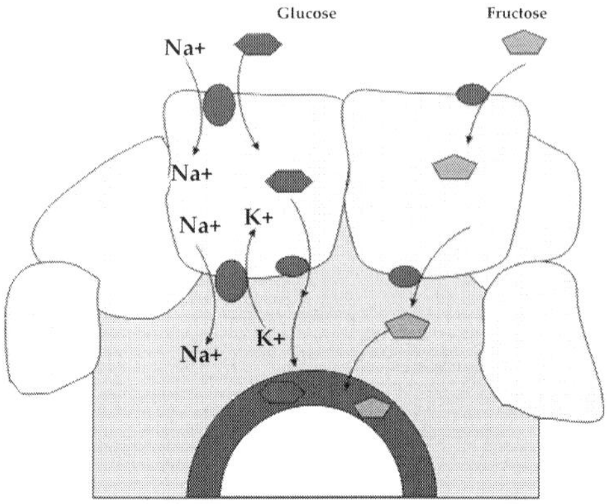

Figure 2.1. Gastrointestinal absorption.

Source: https://upload.wikimedia.org/wikipedia/commons/f/f3/Absorb_sugars.png

2.1.10. Other Routes of Absorption

There are several routes of absorption that are present while conducting experiments related to toxicity, such as intravenous absorption, subcutaneous absorption, intraperitoneal absorption, and intramuscular absorption.

2.1.11. Distribution

The distribution of a chemical compound is a process that occurs within an organism, and this is known to be an active process that largely depends on the uptake and elimination rates of several chemicals. The process of distribution is also dependent on the blood flow and affinity of a particular substance in the blood. Water-soluble, small, uncharged molecules, univalent cations, and most anions diffuse easily and will eventually reach a relatively even distribution in the body.

The distribution of several compounds in the blood is known to be dependent on the Volume of distribution, Accumulation, Barriers in the blood, and Blood binding of the substance.

2.1.12. Elimination

Elimination is the process which is known for the disappearance of a substance in the human body. Elimination of a substance may also refer to the excretion of the chemical compound completely from the body or the transformation of the chemical compound into several other substances. The rate of the disappearance of a chemical substance from the body is known to be mentioned in the form of an elimination rate constant, and is also expressed in the terms of biological half-time or clearance of the compound from the human body.

2.1.13. Excretion

Excretion refers to the elimination or removal or exit of a substance from the human body. This also refers to the biotransformation of products within an organism. The important organs for excretion are kidneys, and several unutilized non-essential products are removed from the body through excretion. The kidneys are the important organs of excretion in the human body. Urine and bile are two important substances that aid in the excretion of a chemical substance from the blood.

A fraction of biliary excreted substances may be reabsorbed in the intestines. This process, enterohepatic circulation, is common for conjugated substances following intestinal hydrolysis of the conjugate.

2.2. BASIC PRINCIPLES OF TOXICOLOGY-FOOD ADDITIVES

2.2.1. Principle 1: Using Toxic Syndrome Recognition for Rapid Diagnosis and Empiric Therapy

The food additives or toxic chemicals are generally grouped into similar classes. These food substances are grouped into several classes because they are known to have similar properties and the same effect on human health.

The chemicals that belong to the same class are known to have similar effects on organisms that are toxic to the living organisms, and these are called toxic effects. Toxic effects are sometimes called toxic syndromes that are known to possess a group of clinical "fingerprints" for a particular class of toxins. Any toxin belonging to a specific group is known to exhibit a similar type of toxic syndromes, and these toxic syndromes are known to be treated similarly.

2.2.1.1. Emergency Treatment

The classes of toxic substances are known to be useful in the case of emergencies and the toxic syndromes that are used in the treatment of people when the exact chemical or food additive that has caused toxicity is unknown. The classes or group of food additives is an extremely useful decision-making tool in the case of an emergency.

There are some basic symptoms are present that are essential in the identification of a toxic syndrome are as follows:

- Vital signs;
- Mental status;
- Pupil size;
- Mucous membrane irritation;
- Lung examination for wheezes or rales;
- Skin for burns, moisture, and colour.

The primary step in the identification and treatment of any toxicity in the human body is generally by a group of signs and symptoms that are necessary to diagnose and treat any life-threatening condition that is caused because of any flavouring agent or additive. The life-threatening condition in the case of any toxicity that is caused because of food additives can be as serious as a respiratory arrest.

The initial treatment of any life-threatening condition will lead to the cure of these symptoms which would later give scope to treat the reaction based on the history or diagnostic test results and some other therapeutic conditions that are exhibited by the patient during treatment. The symptoms and case history would enable the doctor to make decisions regarding the levels of toxicity and influence of toxicity.

2.2.2. Principle 2 Route of Exposure Is a Determinant of Toxicity

The important methodology to determine the mode of toxicity and the influence of toxicity is based on the route of exposure, and some of the important steps in the determination of toxicity are as follows:

- The molecular structure, physical state, and route of exposure to any chemical are known to influence the toxicity of the chemical.
- An important aspect that is related to the toxicity of the chemical is mostly the route of exposure. The route of exposure to the chemical is a great determinant of the toxicity of the chemical.

There are different ways by which the toxicity of the chemical is generally influenced, and the mode of exposure and route of entry of the chemical into the body is the major determining factors of the toxicity of the chemicals. The main reason for the importance of the route of exposure to the chemicals is because many chemicals are known to be absorbed in the site of absorption. The different routes of exposure to the chemical are discussed in the following subsections.

2.2.2.1. Inhalation Exposure

A lot of chemicals are known to enter the system because of inhalation, and the different modes of exposure for inhalation are in the form of gases, vapors, airborne powders, and aerosolized liquids which are known to have toxic effects on the system because of inhalation of these hazardous chemicals into the system.

The inhalation of certain chemicals in the form of gases, vapors, airborne powders is known to be extremely difficult as they would have adverse effects on the respiratory system and would show some sort of toxic effect once it enters into the human body (Figure 2.2).

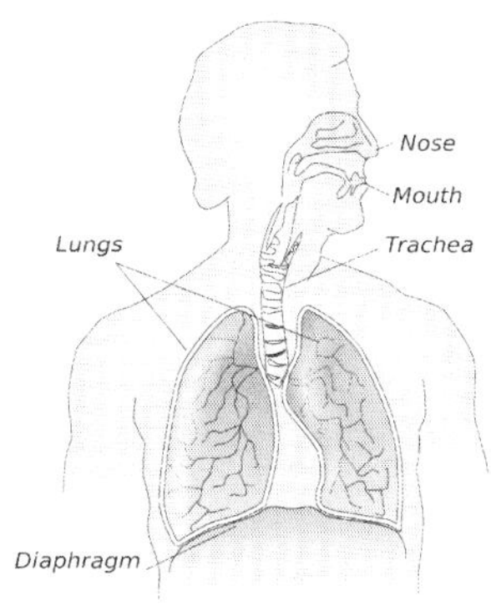

Figure 2.2. Absorption through the nasal system.

Source: https://upload.wikimedia.org/wikipedia/commons/thumb/8/8b/Respiratory_system.svg/2000px-Respiratory_system.svg.png

The different toxic effects of these gases or other chemicals that might have toxic effects are as follows:

- These gases can react with the water in the mucous membranes of the respiratory system, and it can enter the eye while breathing and can cause burning, pain, irritation, and copious secretion at the site of contact or the point of absorption.

- The entry of a toxic chemical through the route of absorption is known to be the quickest way to enter the systemic circulation, and once any chemical enters the systemic circulation, they are known to cause a lot of hazardous effects on the system.
- Hydrogen cyanide is one toxic gas that is extremely hazardous, and it can quickly get absorbed into the circulatory system through inhalation. This gas that is inhaled gets quickly absorbed into the circulatory system through the lungs and is known to cause many toxic effects in individuals.

Some of the consequences of these toxic chemicals entry into the circulatory system are loss of consciousness, seizures, cardiac dysrhythmias, hypotension, and some other effects which may lead to death in a person just minutes after the exposure.

2.2.2.2. Dermal Exposure or Entry of Chemicals through Absorption from Skin

Several chemicals enter the system because of absorption through the skin, and these are absorbed into the system when the person touches or the chemical gets into contact with the skin of the human being. The initial reaction of any of these chemicals is on the skin, and they are known to create allergic reactions in the skin because of exposure to these chemicals. These chemicals are known to cause several toxic effects at the point of contact, and there are cases for these chemicals to enter into the systemic circulation through the absorption from the skin.

Once these chemicals enter the systemic circulation, they are known to create a variety of toxic effects in human beings. The route of exposure is important to understand the toxicity of the chemicals, however, it is important to understand these chemicals not just give allergic reactions or toxic effects at sites that are local to the route of entry, but they are known to create several side effects at places away from the mode of entry in the system.

Some of the chemicals that create toxic effects in human beings after dermal exposure are as follows:

- There are some organophosphate insecticides that are known to be fat-soluble chemicals that can quickly enter into the system through the skin and penetrate the circulatory system. Once these enter the circulatory system, they are known to travel in the blood to different locations and create toxic effects in human beings.

- However, the route of exposure determines the intensity and speed of toxic reactions that can happen in human beings such as the entry of chemicals into the body through the respiratory system can cause severe toxic effects compared to the dermal exposure to the toxic chemicals.

2.2.2.3. Gastrointestinal Absorption

Gastrointestinal absorption is the major route of absorption for any chemicals and area. The food that is consumed generally enters the circulatory system after absorption.

2.2.3. Principle 3: The Dose Makes the Poison

The dosage of the chemicals that are absorbed is known to be an important factor that would determine the response of a particular chemical in the human body. Dose-response refers to a process that is used in diagnosing and understanding the after-effects of exposure to a chemical. The evaluation of the exposure of a chemical, the amount of exposure, and the clinical effects because of exposure is a fundamental principle of toxicology, which is called a dose-response.

The dose-response principle is used predominantly in assessing the clinical effects of any reaction and the different effects based on the dosage of exposure are as follows:

- Dose-response principle helps in understanding, assessing, and evaluating the clinical parameters after exposure.
- Dose refers to the complete amount of the chemical that is absorbed into the system after exposure to the chemical.
- Dose of the chemical is known to be largely dependent on the concentration of the chemical at the time of exposure and the period of exposure, which refers to the period that the chemical is exposed to the human being. The time that the chemical is exposed and the concentration of the chemical are needed to understand the type of toxic effects that are obtained based on the dose.
- An important example of the importance of dosage in the determination of the toxicity of the chemical is Ethanol. The increase of the concentration of ethanol levels in the blood is known to create a gradual increase in alteration of consciousness, poor coordination and may gradually lead to coma and other

respiratory problems such as depression which may slowly lead to the death of the person.

2.2.3.1. Exposure

The exposure of the chemicals to human beings is known to generate toxic effects in human beings. Duration of the exposure to the chemical to the human being is known to be an important factor that can affect the dose of the chemical that enters the circulatory system.

The presence of a greater concentration of a drug and exposure to a higher concentration of the chemical from long periods is known to generate adverse health effects in human beings than the smaller duration of exposure to less concentration of the chemicals. Several instances can explain the period of exposure and dosage of chemicals and how they influence the response to the human beings to these toxic chemicals. Some of the important examples are as follows:

For instance, the dermal exposure of the skin to any acid may cause extreme damage to the skin if the period of exposure of the skin to the acid is high. If the acid is washed off the skin immediately, then the damage that is caused to the skin because of the acid is comparatively less.

There is a similar example to the exposure of the chemical through inhalation, and the exposure through inhalation is known to create rapid adverse reactions in human beings and these are known to be extremely high if there is a higher concentration of gas that is inhaled for a longer duration rather than smaller concentration of the chemical for a smaller duration.

2.2.4. Application of the Dose-Response Principles of Toxicology

The application of these principles of dose-response to toxicology would play an important role in treating the patients who are exposed to harmful chemicals and are showing toxic responses to the exposure to these chemicals.

The patients are known to exhibit severe consequences when the chemicals are exposed to people who ate higher concentrations for longer periods, leading to several harmful adverse reactions in human beings. The people who are exposed to greater doses of these chemicals would need immediate attention and treatment, whereas, patients who are exposed to smaller quantities of the chemicals for smaller duration are known to show lesser side effects or sometimes may remain asymptomatic.

2.3. PRINCIPLES OF FOOD ADDITIVES AND TOXICOLOGY

Flavouring agents are mostly added to food to enhance the appearance and taste of food. The flavouring agents can either be natural flavouring agents or products that are derived from natural products or synthetic flavouring agents. The flavouring agents or foods additives are known to have varying groups of substances which are comprised of different groups of materials which are as follows:

- The flavouring agents are generally synthetic substances that most likely do not appear naturally in food.
- The flavouring agents are those substances that occur naturally and are generally eaten as food.
- Substances that are derived from natural substances, and these substances are not generally consumed as a part of the diet, and they are mostly used for their natural -identical flavours.
- Some flavouring agents are mostly derived from herbs and spices. These herbs and spice-derived flavouring agents are mostly used as nature-identical flavourings.
- Flavouring agents that are derived from several plants and animals and are known to be mostly consumed as food. These agents can either be processed or non-processed. The synthetic equivalents of these agents are mostly used as flavouring agents.

The quantity of the flavouring agents that is added to the food is known to be extremely less, and it is often known that the exposure to these flavouring agents could be extremely less because of which the chances of these flavouring agents to create toxic effects in human beings is known to be extremely placed. The study and research regarding these flavouring agents suggest that these flavours are generally easily metabolized by the system and lead to the formation of harmless end products (FAO/WHO, 1995).

This aspect, which indicates that the exposure to the food additives is known to be extremely low and they are easily metabolized minimizes the need for toxicological testing of several flavouring agents. The metabolic activity of the additives, chemical structure, structure-activity relationship, and the properties of the additives are extremely important in the safety evaluation of the food additives. The safety evaluation of several food additives and flavouring agents is known to face several challenges. It is important to understand that the flavouring agents are consumed in very small quantities, and there are thousands of food additives that are commercially used across the world. The grouping of different flavouring agents or food additives results in nearly 40 categories or groups of flavouring agents. These different groups of flavouring agents indicate the presence of several categories of chemical structures which are known to have several molecular and physical similarities. These different groups of flavouring agents are unique in their taste, and they are known to have a lot of diverse functions and may differ physically and structurally. They may have a lot of diversity in their structural and physical properties, but they are known to have similar metabolization by the human body.

The process of testing different food additives belonging to these 40 categories can be an extremely difficult challenge as it would involve the utilization of several resources and manpower. The safety evaluation of several chemicals is known to utilize the data and information that is present in the intake, absorption, metabolic fate, and toxicity of the chemicals to evaluate the toxicity of these chemicals. Several tests are present to evaluate the toxicity of the additives that are belonging to unique structural groups.

There are several procedures for the safety evaluation of the flavouring agents and the current JECFA procedure for the testing of flavouring agents is known to be first considered and used in 1995. There was a paper that was published based on this procedure by Munro et al. (1999). This procedure of safety assessment and evaluation of flavouring agents was adopted by JECFA in the 46th meeting in 1997, and several modifications were made to this procedure in later times. This procedure is represented in the form of a picture below.

This particular approach is known to imbibe a set of standards that are intended to suggest a procedure for the assessment of flavouring agents in a consistent and timely manner. These standards are framed in a way by which they take into consideration the metabolism, physical features, structure-activity relationship of the additives, and take into consideration the toxic data that are available regarding the additives. There is a number that is assigned to every flavouring agent, which helps in easy identification and sorting of the flavouring agents.

The use of certain standards to design the safety evaluation procedures is extremely useful in segregating several flavouring agents that are commercially available. This segregation makes it extremely helpful in registering the information regarding flavouring agents such as the toxicity information, absence of safety concerns and it is extremely useful in facilitating with the guidance on the nature and the type of information that is required for safety evaluation.

The criteria take advantage of the fact that some flavouring agents occur as normal constituents of mammalian tissues or are metabolized to form such constituents and are then completely metabolized to innocuous end-products, such as carbon dioxide and water.

The flavouring agents with these characteristics, such as their easy metabolism in the system and converted into innocuous end products, such as carbon dioxide and water, are declared to be extremely safe for consumption. The toxicity data are generally used to assess the severity of exposure, and if the dietary exposure is extremely less or high, this information is mostly utilized to understand the consequences of toxic syndromes that are generated because of exposure.

The safety evaluation of food additives without the information on metabolism is known to be carried out based on the toxicity data. The toxicity data is generally used for safety analysis for these unpredicted food additives rather than using dietary exposure.

The food additives that are generally used these days with zero or no toxicity are known to have a dietary exposure value of 1.5 μg/day, which is extremely less and considered safe for consumption. Those additives with an exposure value of less than 1.5 μg/day are declared safe for consumption only if they show no signs of genotoxicity.

The safety evaluation of those additives which have unsolved problems of toxicity is generally not carried out, and there is no standard procedure for the evaluation of these additives. It was noted that a key element of the procedure involves determining whether a flavouring agent and the products of its metabolism are innocuous or endogenous substances.

2.4. PRINCIPLES OF SAFETY EVALUATION IN TOXICOLOGY

The different principles of food toxicology for the safety assessment of the food additives are written in a book titled Toxicological Principles for the Safety Assessment of Direct Food Additives and Colour Additives Used in Food. This book is popularly called the "Redbook," which was published in 1982 (US FDA, 1982).

food is generally obtained by multiplying the dietary concentration of the additive to the complete weight of the food consumed by an individual per day, which is approximately 3000g.

The EDI of food is known to be different for both the direct food additives and indirect food additives. The recommended daily intake of food for direct additives is generally proposed based on the technical applications of the additive.

The approximate EDI of food for every person who consumes the food with additives and the entire population in countries like the United States is generally obtained by the total consumption of the food that is consumed by the people from all the proposed uses of the food with additives is used to generate the EDI of food separately for gender and age group. This information is used to compare the EDI of the food with the ADI and it is used for carrying out the safety assessment for the ingredient.

The objective is to ensure that the EDI of 90% of the population must be less than the ADI of food. Therefore, it is necessary to report and record the maximum concentration of any particular food additive in food and on the human consumption rates of the food item including the 90% of the population must be recorded. The food additive is generally accepted if the EDI of the additive is known to be less than the accepted daily intake of the food additive.

The procedure for the calculation of EDI of food is explained below, and this procedure is explained by Frankos and Rodricks. There are different requirements while calculating the EDI for different nations and the EDI for the entire population of the European Union is mostly for 95%, unlike other countries.

In the performance of the dietary intake assessment if a food additive the concentration of a particular food additive or ingredient in the food is generally found by:

- The approximate use of those ingredients in food at certain levels, which are generally typical, recommended, or maximum.
- The estimated concentration of the food additive that is consumed by the individual after the losses that have happened to the additive because of processing and storing of such ingredients.
- The limit of detection (LOD) or limit of quantification (LOQ) of the analytical method if the concentration of any food ingredient

is known to be nondetectable or nonquantifiable at a given LOD or LOQ.

- The specifications that are set for any particular substance, such as the specifications in the form of CFR or food chemical codex of any particular food which either has unrequired impurities or any other contaminants in the food.
- The list of the levels of the contaminants that are adopted by food are known to have a standard body for setting the limitations of these ingredients in food and the bodies that are used for setting the level of food contaminants are organizations such as the Codex Alimentarius Commission (CAC). The FDA typically uses the maximum intended use levels proposed to calculate a worst-case level of intake.

There are several organizations and multiple bodies that are present to give estimations regarding several food additives and procedures that are present in the toxicity levels that are present in the food additives. Though several organizations are responsible for giving information regarding the several estimations of food additives that are added to food, the most important organizations from which these estimations are obtained are the National Health and Nutrition Examination Survey (NHANES).

The information that is obtained from surveys conducted by these organizations is known to have made the data available publicly to facilitate easy use and make the information useful to everyone. This information from these surveys is known to be extremely beneficial and is considered authentic to use this information.

2.5. CONCLUSION

Toxicology refers to the different types of responses that are generated in living organisms because of the consumption of certain chemicals or synthetic substances. Different types of food additives can be grouped into several categories that are added to the food of living organisms. These food additives can be grouped into several different categories based on their molecular structure and functional properties.

Food additives can be broadly classified into three different categories based on the molecular structure and toxicity of the food. These three categories are category A, Category B, and Category C, where the first category is low toxic, medium toxic, and highly toxic chemicals. There are several principles of safety evaluation of food additives, and these additives are carefully monitored and evaluated for any possible carcinogenic properties.

There is a lot of research that is carried out on these chemicals, and there are certain threshold limits that are standardized for the safe consumption of certain food additives. The safe consumption of food additives has two main constraints called EDI and ADI. There is a need to have the right balance between the EDI and the ADI where the EDI needs to be maintained across the consumption of several food substances.

The food additive that enters the system is generally absorbed by the gastrointestinal tract and enters into the circulatory system. The additives generally are metabolized to produce innocuous end products that generate just water and carbon dioxide. Food additives are generally naturally derived flavouring agents or synthetically derived food substances. There is an allowed threshold for the consumption of these food substances, and if they are consumed in huge amounts, they lead to adverse drug reactions in human beings.

The effect of these substances is generally dependent on two factors, such as the period of exposure and the concentration of exposure. If the period of exposure or the concentration of the exposure of any food substance is known to be high then there is a greater risk of toxic response, whereas minimal exposure would lead to less toxic effects or reaction in human beings.

The dose-effect and dose-response curves are known to be an essential aspect of any toxicological evaluation of drugs or chemicals. Each chemical compound can have different types of drug response curves at the level of a cell, tissues, organ, and organism.

Several stages are present in the safety evaluation of the drugs, and it is important to understand the levels of concern of different additives. There are three levels of concerns that are important for any additives, and these are dependent on the toxicity, chemical structure of these additives.

REFERENCES

1. FAO (2019). Food Safety and Quality: Guidelines. [online] Fao.org. Available at: http://www.fao.org/food/food-safety-quality/scientific-advice/jecfa/guidelines0/en/ (Accessed on 14 May 2019).
2. Pressman, P., Reddy, C., Clemens, R., & Hayes, W., (2017). Food Additive Safety: A Review of Toxicologic and Regulatory Issues. [online] Journals.sagepub.com. Available at: https://journals.sagepub.com/doi/pdf/10.1177/2397847317723572 (Accessed on 14 May 2019).
3. Who, W., (2019). Principles and Methods for the Risk Assessment of Chemicals in Food. [online] Inchem.org. Available at: http://www.inchem.org/documents/ehc/ehc/ehc240_chapter9.pdf (Accessed on 14 May 2019).
4. who.int (2019). Principles and Methods for the Risk Assessment of Chemicals in Food. [online] Who.int. Available at: https://www.who.int/foodsafety/chem/special_considerations.pdf (Accessed on 14 May 2019).

Chapter 3

Food Additives and Food Acidulants

CONTENTS

Food additives and acidulants are widely used to improve the texture, flavor, and appearance of food and enhance their shelf-life. This chapter discusses the reasons for their usage and the acceptable daily intake (ADI) of food additives. It then covers the function and usage of additives in the food industry. There are various types of food additives and acidulants used in the food industry, which the chapter elucidates. Finally, it covers the global regulation for food additives and the "big three" regulations.

3.1. INTRODUCTION

Additives are utilized to improve food. They can:

- Improve the keeping nature of food by making it keep going longer on the rack or in the cooler, for instance, an additive to forestall the development of microbes or a humectant to prevent food from drying out;
- Improve the taste or presence of food, for instance, by the utilization of flavors, thickeners, and hues.

Another advantage of food additives is that shoppers can be offered a more extensive selection of foods. Many handled foods contain additives. Some regular models are bacon, margarine, frozen yogurt, and bread. A few people trust that since food additives are synthetic chemicals, they ought to be prohibited. However, everything on the planet, including us and the food we eat, is made of synthetic concoctions.

Air, water, glucose, and salt are synthetic additives; similar to what food additives are. Numerous food additives happen normally, for example, red shading from beetroot (Beet red), and purple shading from grape skins (anthocyanins).

These hues can be removed and to foods. Some food additives found in nature can be produced, for instance, ascorbic chemicals. Different additives are produced but not found in nature, for example, aspartame, which is utilized to supplant sugar.

Controlling the utilization of additives before an additive can be utilized in foods; Food Standards Australia New Zealand (FSANZ) does a wellbeing evaluation. All additives experience a wellbeing evaluation process. FSANZ watches that the food additive is sheltered at the dimension proposed to be utilized and that there are great innovative explanations behind the utilization of the additive. If FSANZ concurs that a food additive ought to be allowed, endorsement of government ministers is looked for. It is simply after Ministerial endorsement that a food additive can be utilized in foods. The Food Standards Code (this is the joint food law among Australia and New Zealand) says which additives can be utilized and in what foods. Additives and unfavourable responses (Intolerance, sensitivities) few individuals may have unfriendly responses to some food additives, similarly as certain individuals might be susceptible to or have antagonistic responses to peanuts, milk, or shellfish.

Food naming helps individuals who are touchy to certain food additives to maintain a strategic distance from them. Perusing the food name to check what additives are in foods, read the mark. All food fixings, including any additives, must be recorded in the name of the food.

The fixings are recorded in slipping request of ingoing weight. On the name, inside the rundown of fixings, the class name of the additive will be recorded and after that the additive name or code number in sections. For instance:

- Thickener (gelatin); or
- Thickener, (440).

3.1.1. Class Name

Food additives are gathered into classes as indicated by their capacity. For instance, all shading additives are utilized to shading food, so are in one gathering in this booklet. Some food additives have more than one use. It's just plain obvious, for instance, Soy Lecithin (number 322). It tends to be utilized as a cell reinforcement, and as an emulsifier. It consequently has two passages in this booklet. Where an additive is fit for being ordered in more than one class, the most suitable class name is utilized on the mark of a food.

Now and again there are discretionary or elective class names not recorded in this booklet that can be utilized in the name. For instance, a few thickeners can also be called changed starches. A few additives don't have a legitimately characterized class name. The gathering of additives that work as charges (see the table in this booklet) has no lawfully characterized class name, so are recorded in the name by the particular name of the additive, with no reference to a class name.

3.1.2. Code Numbers

Most food additives have code numbers. The numbers recorded in this booklet are a piece of a worldwide numbering framework. Code numbers utilize less space on marks than names of additives. They also help stay

CASE STUDY

Why Do We Use Additives?

Additives serve a wide variety of uses. For example, preservatives protect foods against deterioration and prevent growth of fungi and bacteria. Other additives help improve the texture and consistency of foods, keep them flowing freely when poured, or prevent them from drying out. Flavorings restore taste losses or can enhance the flavor or aroma of food. Emulsifiers ensure that oil and water in foods do not separate. According to FSANZ, additives serve three purposes:

- Improve the taste or appearance of a processed food;
- Improve the keeping quality or stability of a food; and
- Preserve food when this is the most practical way of extending its storage life.

Are All Additives Artificial?

Many additives have unpronounceable or complex chemical names. It is often assumed that long chemical names indicate that an additive is artificial. This is not always true. Take the following list of ingredients:

- Acetaldehyde;
- Ethanol;
- Propan-1-ol;
- Ethyl pentanoate;
- Ethyl hexanoate;
- Ethyl-2-methyl butanoate;
- 2 methyl butyl acetate.

These are just a few of the chemicals that flavor an apple, many natural and commonly occurring products are used as food additives. Salt, sugar, vinegar, and some vitamins are used as preservatives. Many food colorings and flavorings are obtained from foods. The food additive 300 is vitamin C; 101 is Vitamin B2 (riboflavin), and grape skin extract has the number 163.

Safety and Dose

The use of food additives in Australia is regulated by Food Standard Australia and New Zealand (FSANZ). FSANZ does not approve an additive unless extensive testing has been undertaken and it has been shown that no harmful effects are expected from consumption. For a chemical to be approved it must be demonstrated that it is safe, there are good reasons to use it, it will be used in the lowest possible quantity and that consumers will be clearly informed when it is added (through Labeling). 1 FSANZ also sets the ADI for each additive – that is, the amount that can be eaten every day over a lifetime without risk of harm. The ADI is determined by reviewing available data and finding a level at which no toxic effect is observed. A large safety factor is included in the ADI, which means that the level at which no toxic effect is observed is multiplied, often by more than 100, to produce the ADI. 1 FSANZ also estimate the expected daily intake – how much an average person is likely to consume of the chemical from the food supply.

This assessment is compared to the ADI and determines how much of the chemical can be added to food. The expected daily intake is modified in response to changes in food consumption patterns. For example, when FSANZ found that 5% of children in between the ages of 2 and 11 years were consuming more than the expected daily intake of an artificial sweetener named cyclamate, they reduced the maximum amount allowed in flavored drinks by almost half. 1 Many consumers are not comforted by the fact that they are eating an ingredient at a fraction of the level at which it causes observable toxic effects. Some argue that an ingredient with ANY toxic effects at ANY level should be avoided. It is worth noting that chemicals which are necessary at lower levels, such as salt or vitamin A, can be extremely harmful if the dose taken is too high.

Controversial Additives

1. ***Monosodium Glutamate (MSG):*** Or 621 are often added to food as a flavor enhancer. The sodium component is identical to sodium from table salt. Glutamate is an amino acid – the building block of protein – that is found in many proteins that are commonly eaten. MSG occurs naturally in many protein-rich foods, and is harvested from sugar cane for use as a food additive. 3 FSANZ conducted a thorough safety assessment of MSG (or 621).

In this assessment, MSG was explored as a possible cause of Chinese restaurant syndrome and asthmatic attacks. Symptoms of Chinese restaurant syndrome include numbness, weakness, drowsiness, nausea, and headache. Evidence remains inconclusive, and the studies which do establish a link suggest that it only exists for a small percentage of the population. Evidence for the link between asthma and MSG is also inconclusive, because results from different studies conflict.

Animal studies indicate that the ADI for MSG is 16,000 mg (16 grams) per kilo of body weight per day (mg/kg/day). A report published in the European Journal of Clinical Nutrition suggests that amongst extreme users of MSG, intake is 30 mg/kg/day, which is well within the ADI. The same report reviewed a study in which humans were given doses of free glutamate of 147 grams a day or more, without any adverse effects. Extreme users of MSG are thought to consume 2–3 grams of MSG a day.

2. ***Sodium Nitrate and Sodium Nitrit***e: Nitrites and nitrates are used as a preservative and add color and flavor to processed meats. Processed meats are those meats that are commonly eaten cold and are pink or red in color. The International Agency for the Research of Cancer (IARC) has reviewed ingested nitrates and nitrites and classified them as 'probably carcinogenic to humans' by the IARC. Nitrites and nitrates have been linked to bowel cancer, one of the most common cancers in men and women in Australia.

3.4. TYPES OF ADDITIVES IN PROCESSED FOODS

Processed food manufacturers often claim that there are "no additives or preservatives added" in the food labels. However, it is hard-pressed to find any product in a supermarket which does not contain at least one additive. Even products that claim to be organic have at least one additive added to them. The only way, in this modern world to avoid additives is by making food from the scratch.

Essentially, food additives are natural, nature-identical, and artificial ingredients that are added to food. The purpose of adding them is to improve flavour, appearance, and increase their shelf life. Some natural additives were being used since historical times, for example, salt to cure meat. In the 20th century, advances in chemical and food engineering brought endless innovations in additives, resulting in the products currently lining supermarket shelves all around the globe. Many of these additives are harmful to health, while some have been recognized as safe to consume. A thorough understanding of the additives helps in identifying the additives which are toxic to the body. The additives can be roughly categorized into the following types. Some additives belong to more than one category. For instance, salt is both a flavour enhancer and a preservative.

3.4.1. Preservatives

Preservatives are perhaps the most widely used additive which is used in almost all processed foods. It increases their shelf life by preventing spoilage from bacteria, fungi, and viruses. There are three natural preservatives, salt, sugar, and vinegar. Salt is used as a preservative in Indian pickles. Vinegar is used in pickled mango, jalapeno, etc. Sugar is used in jams. Salt and sugar extract water from the microorganisms and inhibit their growth. Vinegar maintains an acidic condition where microbes cannot survive.

However, artificial flavours are more in use in processed food. Nitrates and nitrites are used in meat, burger, and sausages. Sulphur dioxide is used in fruit juice. Home-baked bread has a shelf life of 36 hours, where store-bought ones last a week due to the presence of propionates which inhibit mold formation.

These preservatives have adverse health effects. Nitrite added to meat, produce nitrosamines during cooking, which can cause cancer. Sulphur dioxide can trigger asthma and allergies in certain people.

3.4.2. Sweeteners

Sugar and high fructose corn syrup (HFCS) are some ‘natural sweeteners. It is found in high amounts in juice, candy, soda, cereals, and snacks. Fructose is a simple sugar that harms the body, including diabetes, obesity, tooth decay, etc. It causes a significant increase in belly fat and increases blood sugar levels and decreased insulin sensitivity. Studies conducted in animals reveal that fructose can cause cell inflammation. This can lead to many chronic conditions like diabetes, heart attack, and cancer. Moreover, they have no nutritional value and simply increase calorie intake.

There are many artificial sweeteners available, which are mainly used in diet food and consumed by weight watchers and diabetics. They are used in food and beverage to enhance sweetness without adding calories. Some low-calorie sweeteners include sucralose, aspartame, acesulfame potassium, and saccharin.

The effects of artificial sweeteners have been studied for decades. Critics argue that they lead to many health problems, including cancer. In the 1970s, the use of saccharin caused cancer in rats. However, the National Cancer Institute and other health agencies have not found any scientific links between artificial sweeteners and cancer or other health issues. Many studies concluded that it was safe even for women.

3.4.3. Antioxidant

Foods that have oils and fat can become rancid. The fats and oils get oxidized when exposed to air, and they emit an unpleasant odor. Many foods oxidize when they come in contact with air, like apples and potatoes. Antioxidants are added to food so that fats do not become rancid, and fruits do not turn brown.

The use of antioxidants BHA and BHT harmed dogs and hence has been controversial. The safest antioxidants known are vitamin C, and vitamin E. Vitamin C has many health benefits, including preventing cancer and enhancing the immunity system. Vitamin E reduces the risk of heart diseases and cancer by neutralizing free radicals. Sodium citrate is used in cooked cured meat to prevent fats from turning rancid. Frozen foods have antioxidants, which reduce the deterioration rate of these foods and keep them fresh for longer.

3.4.4. Acids

They are added to food to make flavor sharper. It also has preservative properties and antioxidants. Some of the acids used in food are vinegar, ascorbic acid, and citric acid. Acids have been used to counteract pathogenic microorganisms for decades; however, there is a need to evaluate their effectiveness and suitability and improve them. There is also increased awareness about the negative effects of these acids, and hence, there is a growing demand to use milder treatments to preserve foods.

Is a weak carboxylic acid. It occurs naturally in fruits. It has been added to processed food for over a century. It occurs in many of the food and drink products and is listed under its E number, E330. It plays a significant role in the food processing industry since it is versatile in its use.

Organic acids are now gaining popularity because it concentrates on safe and effective techniques for applying organic acids for the prevention of bacterial growth. There is a wide range of potentially useful antimicrobials, and only a few can be used for practical purposes.

3.4.5. Anticaking Agent

Anticaking agents are food additives that maintain the free flow of powders and granulated materials by preventing their agglomeration. Products that use anticaking agents are milk powder, coffee powder, powdered sugar that is used in coffee machines. They prevent the formation of lumps, making it suitable for packing, transporting, and final consumption.

Anticaking agents absorb the extra moisture or make the food particles water repellent. Some of these additives are soluble in water, others in alcohol or organic solvents. Some additives absorb both salt and oil like Calcium silicate ($CaSiO_3$), which is added to salt. Sodium bicarbonate is another popular anticaking agent.

Anticaking agents can be natural or manufactured. Most of them contain synthetic substances like silicon dioxide or magnesium and calcium stearates (solid saturated fatty acids.). There are some which come from nature like kaolin (E559; talc (E553b); and bentonite. Organic and hypoallergenic anticaking agents are made from natural products like rice (Figure 3.2).

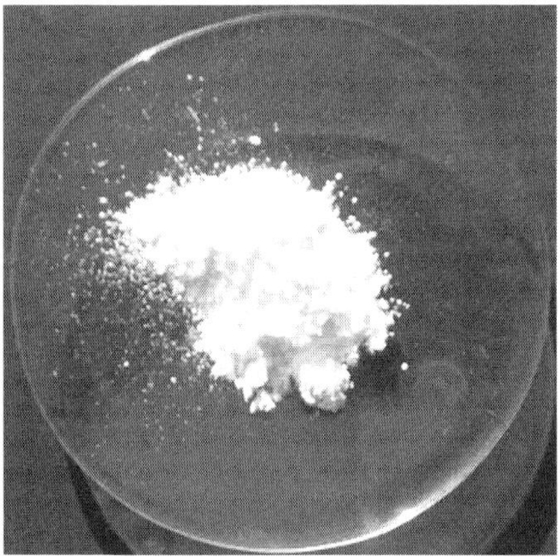

Figure 3.2. Representation of anticaking agent.

Source: https://upload.wikimedia.org/wikipedia/commons/thumb/1/13/Magnesium_oxide.jpg/621px-Magnesium_oxide.jpg

3.4.6. Bulking Agents

These additives increase the volume of the food but contain no nutritional value. They promote a sense of satiety and are hence commonly used in diet foods aimed at weight loss. It does not alter the taste of the food and hence

3.4.10. Flavours

Flavours, both natural and artificial, are added to food to enhance its taste and aroma. They are added to food to restore taste that is lost during processing. While natural flavours are safe and may also have certain health benefits, the same cannot be said for artificial flavours. Artificial flavours are chemicals that mimic the taste of natural substances or add their taste. Artificial flavours can imitate many natural flavours like caramel, fruit, spices, etc. Some examples of artificial flavours are MSG, which is used in frozen food, salad dressings, spice mixes, etc. It is also used in food preparation in Chinese restaurants.

Research reveals that artificial flavours can have an adverse impact on health. Red cell production in rats dropped drastically when artificial colours were fed regularly. Flavours like chocolate, strawberries also have a toxic effect on the body. Similarly, artificial fruit flavours inhibited cell division and damaged the bone marrow cells in mice. However, more research is required in this field to establish the effects of these additives on the body.

3.5. TYPES OF ACIDS AND ACIDULANTS

Acidulants impart a sharp taste to food. They also extend the shelf life of the food products. The pH of a food is a measure of its acidity, alkalinity, or neutrality. Many foods are naturally acidic like oranges, lemons, tomatoes, yogurt. They contain citric acid that imparts a sharp taste.

Acids and alkalis are important to the food industry. Acids have been used for centuries to enhance the flavour of food and prevent microbial growth. Bicarbonates like soda are mild alkalis. Phosphates are used as buffers, besides their characteristic tastes. In the modern-day, the food industry makes use of acidulants. The most organic acid is citric acid. It is widely used in the food, beverage, and pharmaceutical industry.

Commonly used acids and acidulants in food processing are discussed below.

3.5.1. Citric Acid

Citric acid is the most commonly used acid in making beverages. In ancient times, citric acid was derived from limes and lemons. At present, it is produced commercially by a fermentation process. It is used in sweets, cold drinks, jellies, desserts, and various other foods (Figure 3.4).

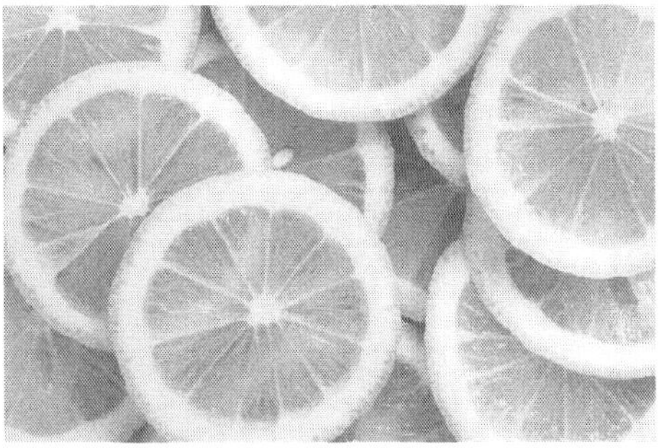

Figure 3.4. Lemon is a significant source of citric acid.

Source: https://cdn.pixabay.com/photo/2018/10/25/08/56/acid-3771954_960_720.jpg

3.5.2. Acetic Acid

Food-grade acetic acid is found in vinegar. It has a pungent taste and is used extensively in the pickling industry. The fermented vinegar naturally has variable pH, and thus, food-grade acetic acid is used for creating pickling liquor that has a specified acidity. It is also used in flavourings and confectionary items.

3.5.3. Fumaric Acid

This food acidulant has a sharp taste. It is not very soluble, which limits its usage in food and drinks processing. It is used in cheesecake mixes, and dessert mixes having gelatin and other beverage powders. Fumaric acid is reasonably priced, and hence, it is also good for making animal feeds.

3.5.4. Lactic Acid

Lactic acid is widely for making pickled foods and boiled sweets. Emulsifiers contain lactic acid, which is used for baking purposes. It can be produced naturally by fermentation. However, most chemical manufacturing companies use synthetically produced lactic acid.

3.5.5. Phosphoric Acid

Phosphoric acid is the second most used acidulant in the food and beverage industry. It is used in cola drinks which have high global sales. It has harsh, biting tastes which add a nice flavour to coal drink.

3.5.6. Malic Acid

Malic acid occurs naturally in apples, tomatoes, cherries, bananas, etc. It is used in the beverage industry for making low-calorie drinks. It is similar in application to citric acid but is slightly expensive than it.

3.5.7. Tartaric Acid

Tartaric acid was widely used in the past; however, it has now been replaced by citric acid. The most common use is as bread improver emulsifiers. It occurs naturally and can be manufactured synthetically as well.

3.6. GLOBAL REGULATION OF FOOD ADDITIVES

U.S food safety laws were concerned with the use of food additives for over a century. The regulation of food additives globally has been led for many decades by the three most robust and distinct safety assessment programs currently in place as well as their predecessor organizations. The big three are:

- The JECFA;
- The European Union Scientific Committee on Food is now known as the European Food Safety Authority (EFSA); and
- United States FDA.

The world today is more aware of the need for consistent regulations in the areas of food additives. Consequently, many countries are trying to establish robust premarket clearance and labeling requirements for them. Countries that do not have well-developed regulatory programs rely on the past reviews of the big three for the assessment process.

Many systems that are still evolving use the big three as a basis, while considering that some cultural differences may not be compatible with these standards. GSFA overtime may make all the national standards uniform so that the food safety of the global supplies chain can be assessed using a unified approach.

3.6.1. United States Regulation of Food Additives/Ingredients

The US regulation is a complex one. The way US law defines food additives is different from the definitions used by EFSA, Codex, and the GSFA in some significant ways. It excludes colour additives and includes indirect additives. As a result, the U.S. is unique in regulating components of food contact materials as "indirect" food additives and in regulating food colours separately from other food ingredients/additives. It also exempts certain substances that were in use 1958.

The major point of difference is that in the US, there is a unique exemption from premarket approvals for using substances that are certified as safe by experts. The GRAS exemption permits safety based on common use before 1958 or on scientific assessment similar to other food substances. This implies that the GRAS uses of food substances are not bound by FDA authorization and listing. As per this regulation, GRAS status would consider the same quantity and quality of information that is required to assess whether food additive is safe.

The data used must be available easily and accepted by all. If either general availability or general acceptance is not fulfilled, the food ingredient has to be premarket reviewed by FDA and includes a full safety assessment. If FDA judges the use of the additive to be safe, then FDA is required to promulgate a regulation in 21 CFR permitting the intended use of the additive and including any specifications and limitations necessary to ensure safe use of the additive.

3.6.2. Safety Assessment of Food Additives

The FDA's assessment is mainly concerned with two questions:

- Is there sufficient data available on toxicity to address concerns regarding the safe consumption of food additives? and
- Do those data reliably convey the safety of the potential exposure to these additives?

The first question can be answered considering the relevant testing recommendations. The process followed by FDA does not have a rigid requirement for the types of testing to be used. It adopts a general approach to evaluate whether the toxicity data is adequate. If a specific study is found necessary to ensure safe use, more assessments will be required in accordance with relevant regulations, guidelines, and standard practice.

The next part of the FDA's toxicity assessment involves the actual evaluation of toxicity testing data. FDA reviewers typically receive and examine the raw data in toxicity studies to arrive at their conclusions regarding the results including any adverse effects, no adverse effect levels (NOAEL), low effect levels, and other positive or negative indications for toxicological concern.

NOAEL can be established from the relevant toxicological data. In the past, FDA would apply an appropriate safety factor to NOAEL to arrive at the ADI.

However, recently, ADI is not used much; instead, the decisions are based on the difference between NOAEL and estimated dietary exposure. The risk management decision of whether or not to permit a food additive would take into consideration whether the estimated dietary exposure is less than ADI. Another parameter is whether estimated dietary exposure is at a much lower level than NOAEL.

In cases where the dietary exposure is extremely low, and a NOAEL is not possible to derive is generally not required to establish safety. IT is common to reference the dietary exposure at which additional data might be recommended as a substitute for the ADI for the additive if short-term testing does not suggest a need for testing on which a NOAEL might be based. These circumstances entail risk management decisions based on long-term toxicity testing data.

3.6.3. EFSA Regulation of Food Additives

The EFSA's framework is similar to the U.S process concerning data requirement and data review. The different EU nations have different consumption patterns and supporting data. As a result, it can lead to higher estimated consumer exposure based on the food additive used. There is no major difference between the US and the EU process of approval of food additives. The EFSA frameworks include food colour within the definition of food additives. However, it does not include processing aids.

EFSA mandates that all food additives used must be on the EFSA listing and should be authorized for use. Commonly used foods like salt sugar do not require premarket approval. Even though processing aids do not require premarket approval, manufacturers have to assess whether they are safe under the general standard.

Essentially, how processing aid is treated is similar to the FDA's implementation of GRAS, though its scope is more limited. One major difference between the US and EU processes is that EFSA explicitly states the cyclic reconsideration of the safety of additives. EU also requires that food additives should be listed in the relevant legislation post the safety assessment. The European Commission is responsible for adding additives to these regulations. Five regulations at present govern the usage of food additives:

- EU 1330/2008 (Common Procedures);
- EU 231/2012 (Specifications and Limitations);
- EU 1333/2008 (Approved Food Additives);
- EU 1334/2008 (Approved Food Flavours); and
- EU 1332/2008 (Approved Food Enzymes).

3.6.4. International Review and Standard-Setting Bodies

The CCFA has worked since the mid-1990s to develop the GSFA to integrate food additive standards with the Codex Alimentarius food standards. Another purpose is to provide a clear recommendation for using food additives that have been identified by JECFA as safe to use. JECFA was founded with the support of the Codex Alimentarius Commission (CAC). The aim was to assess the levels of risk associated with using food additives in food.

JECFA gathers experts from various countries to participate in the assessment of food additives. The methodology adopted by JECFA for assessing dietary exposure and the potential level of toxicity is followed by US FDA and EFSA programs mentioned in the EHC 240: Principles and methods for the risk assessment of chemicals in food. Additives that JECFA considers safe for consumption, JECFA, in most cases, propose specifications concerning identity purity and the use of food additives for adoption by the CCFA.

CCFA meets as a group of delegations of member states as well as delegations for other interested organizations which provide technical support to the GSFA working group and to the CCFA. The annual review of JECFA is conducted by CCFA, which may add further provisions in GSFA if it deems necessary. To date, 46 meetings have been conducted by CCFA, wherein more than 300 food additive provisions have been added to GSFA, and more than 2000 provisions related to additives that are being used are pending incorporation.

Besides implementing the current provisions, the CCFA may seek access to further review and information by JECFA. This is about those specifications that are not adopted for newly proposed food additive uses or for review of food additives for which significant new safety data or new safety questions have come to light.

REFERENCES

1. A Plus Topper, (2017). Types of Food Additives and Their Functions – A Plus Topper. [online] Available at: https://www.aplustopper.com/types-food-additives-functions/ (Accessed on 14 May 2019).
2. Ahu Matua, M., (n.d.). Identifying Food Additives. [eBook] Ministry of primary industries. Available at: https://www.hawkinswatts.com/wp-content/uploads/2016/02/7138896-2013-MPI-Identifying-Food-Additives.pdf (Accessed on 14 May 2019).
3. Branen, L., Davidson, M., Salmien, S., & Thorngate, J., (n.d.). Food Additives (2nd edn.). [eBook] Available at: http://ariefm.lecture.ub.ac.id/files/2012/10/A._Larry_Branen_P._Michael_Davidson_Seppo_SalmiBookFi.org-FOOD-ADDITIVES.pdf (Accessed on 14 May 2019).
4. Cancer Myths (2019). [eBook] Cancer Council, Western Australia. Available at: https://www.cancerwa.asn.au/resources/2013-02-01-food-additives-and-cancer.pdf (Accessed on 14 May 2019).
5. Cheeseman, M., (2019). Global Regulation of Food Additives. [eBook] Available at: https://pubs.acs.org/doi/pdf/10.1021/bk-2014-1162.ch001 (Accessed on 14 May 2019).
6. Food Additives (2012). [eBook] International Dairy Federation. Available at: https://www.fil-idf.org/wp-content/uploads/2016/04/Food-additives.pdf (Accessed on 14 May 2019).
7. Foodadditivesworld.com., (n.d.). Anticaking Agents, Anti Caking Agents, Natural Anticaking Agents, Natural Anti Caking Agents. [online] Available at: http://www.foodadditivesworld.com/anticaking-agents.html (Accessed on 14 May 2019).
8. Fooducate.com., (2011). 11 Types of Food Additives. [online] Available at: https://www.fooducate.com/community/post/11%20Types%20of%20Food%20Additives/57A33CB9-B82E-3993-4F43-BFE94A162EBE (Accessed on 14 May 2019).
9. monarchchemicals.co.uk., (2018). The Role of Citric Acid in the Food & Drink Industry. [online] Available at: https://www.monarchchemicals.co.uk/Information/News-Events/440-/The-Role-of-Citric-Acid-in-the-Food-amp-Drink-Industry (Accessed on 14 May 2019).
10. Pubs.acs.org., (2019). [online] Available at: https://pubs.acs.org/doi/pdf/10.1021/bk-2014-1162.ch001 (Accessed on 14 May 2019).
11. Theron, M. M., & Lues, J., (2010). Organic Acids and Food Preservation.

[online] CRC Press. Available at: https://www.crcpress.com/Organic-Acids-and-Food-Preservation/Theron-Lues/p/book/9781420078428 (Accessed on 14 May 2019).

12. Thomas, S., (2016). 7 Popular Acids and Acidulants Use in Food and Beverage Industry. [online] Medium. Available at: https://medium.com/@stanleythomas.usa/7-popular-acids-and-acidulants-use-in-food-and-beverage-industry-b4b052883acc (Accessed on 14 May 2019).
13. Zelman, K., (2017). Food Additives: Emulsifiers | Food & Nutrition | November-December 2017. [online] Food & Nutrition Magazine. Available at: https://foodandnutrition.org/november-december-2017/food-additives-emulsifiers/ (Accessed on 14 May 2019).

Chapter 4

Natural Toxins in Plant and Animal Stuffs

CONTENTS

This chapter talks about

- The natural toxins present in plants and their products.
- The toxins present in our food and its various types and how they can harm the bodies.
- The toxins present in animals which get build up after some toxins passed from plants to animals as the toxins, which animal's bodies produce which are harmful to human bodies if they consume them as meat.
- The effects of synthetic and organic toxins have on human bodies that are present in our food.
- The various types of toxins present in plants and animals.

4.1. INTRODUCTION

4.1.1. The Natural Toxins in Food

The toxins are inside as natural elements in our food, as opposite of synthetic chemicals or medicines used in plants like pesticides, drugs for animals, or as contaminants present in nature. The natural contaminants are deadly for animals and people who are inside the plants if consumed in satisfactory quantities.

4.1.2. The Origin of Food

Plants and animals produce a variety of contaminants. The natural contaminants inside the plants and animals can be there for a particular task or have transformed as chemical weapons against attackers, insects, or microorganisms. The chemicals have different chemical structures and are extremely different in nature and toxicity.

4.1.3. Natural Toxins Present in Food of Plant Origin

There are over three lakh diverse types of plants varieties present in the world and from which a minimum of over two lakhs are thought to be poisonous. The people and animals if accidentally eat these wild varieties of mushrooms, berries, or other plants they can get poisoned. The plants world over are eaten in hundreds, and many can become poison for the body if consumed in large quantities or not properly washed before being eaten. The parts eaten are different in each variety and it may contain foliage, buds, stems, roots, fruits, and tubers, and so are their poisonous parts.

The plants belonging to the same variety show the same or vastly different toxicities. The quantity and the circulation of the contaminants contained in a plant differ rendering to the species as well as the geographical conditions where it originates.

Normally the flowers and seeds will store defense chemicals and are necessary organs for continued life and reproduction. These contaminants can be very fastly produced or stored at many different stages of important growth that is in the bottom of flowers, young tissue, or seedlings as in the case of potato sprouts.

The most shared examples of natural contaminants in food plants contain glycoalkaloids in potatoes, elements that give birth to cyanide in unpleasant apricot seeds and bamboo shoots, enzyme inhibitors and lectins in soya beans, green beans, and other pulses plants.

4.1.4. Natural Toxins Present in Food of Animal Origin

The natural contaminants of origin of animals are the product digestive process or chemicals; that is coming come from the food chain. The land animals if consumed the cases of poisoning are common, the contamination due to sea poison happens in many parts of the world. The microalgae produce different types of contaminants and it gets deposited in shellfish, crustacean, and finfish following their consumption. The type of bacteria produces tetrodotoxin, a strong marine neurotoxin.

It is found in over 90 species of pufferfish and may cause lethality after ingesting even a small amount. The coral reef fish if eaten then poisoning case is common as it contains ciguatoxin that might be found in more than 300 species of fish. The different type of poisoning due to seafood is by spoiling due to bacteria the histamine is produced in scombroid fish causes a different type of seafood poisoning.

There are about 1200 varieties of toxic and noxious animals in the world. The animals mostly are not consumed or reared as food, but caution is necessary to throw out the contaminating body part and glands containing the poison when these animals are used as food. People eat glands of insects or animals which are thought as safe to consume but these glands contain chemicals like the gall-bladder of grass carp which contains cyprinol related chemicals.

4.1.5. Toxic Effects and Food Poisoning

The natural poison that is contained in food can cause significant health problems and damage and conditions like a terminal disease. The important indicators of damage to the body are of different types like normal stomach disturbance, nervous system problem, and respiratory paralysis to fatality. This is a common occurrence that can happen probably in the likely groups of the population such as children and old people.

The indications are mostly visible in one hour or longer or in a few minutes after consumption of different types of sea contaminants in shellfish and other seafood. Severe poisoning is also observed in ingestion of wild mushrooms or not properly washed plants such as ginkgo seeds and bitter apricot seeds. The severe contamination is mostly observed in poisoning started by plants contaminants such as many alkaloids.

Regular consumption will cause poisoning in the liver due to Pyrrolizidine alkaloids that are present in weeds in crops and in certain plants. The poisoning by food depends on the level of poison and the capacity of the body of individual patients.

4.1.6. Risk Reduction Measures

The poison can be decreased in greater amount by proper cooking and doing good processing of food by employing latest techniques. The consumption can be reduced in cases when decreasing the consumption is not possible. The proper cooking of food decreases enzyme inhibitors and lectins of beans. The proper washing, boiling in water, and soaking the eatables also eliminate some cyanide-producing compounds in the foods concerned.

The poison stored in tissues can be eliminated by the removal of gonads, skin, and parts of certain fish. Normally an element will cause how much damage depends on the level of viscosity, the quantity consumed and the health level of the person as the human body can purify our body of a small amount of poison.

Generally, the human being should practice the old conventional ways of purifying the food by practicing the ways known to us from ancient times and try to eat a balanced and variety of food so that our body exposure to certain types of natural toxins can be kept to a safe level.

4.2. NATURAL TOXINS IN FOOD

The living beings' bodies produce chemicals or contaminants and these are known as natural poisons. These types of chemicals are not harmful to the creature which has produced them but it can cause damage to the other living things such as humans if they are consumed. These types of chemical elements have a variety of shapes and their working is different and the level of poison also varies.

There are plants found in nature that can manufacture natural elements and they are toxic to our human bodies if ingested for example, under specific situations, small algae that are not visible from normal human eyes and look like small plants in the ocean can manufacture elements that are lethal to humans but not to shellfish that eat these algae. The shellfish that has contaminants inside its body if eaten as a consequence illness can happen fastly.

Some contaminants are manufactured by plants as a natural resistance system against predators, insects, or microorganisms, or as a result of infection with microorganisms, such as mold, to fight climatic situations like scarcity of water or dangerous humidity.

The natural poison can also germinate from biological systems which are different from whom in which they are found.

There are three important sources:

- The freshly produced parts of plants can become poisonous if they are mixed with lethal non-nutritive plant variety;
- The fresh meat or matter of animals, mostly fish and milk, can also become dirty if the animal has consumed poisonous matter of natural origin; and
- The microorganisms can manufacture poison of natural origin.

The ingestion of poisonous cereals has caused many cases reported as lethal contamination. The main elements which are responsible are pyrrolizidine alkaloids, manufactured by the genera Senecio, Crotalaria, and Heliotropium (Figure 4.1).

The chemicals responsible for severe liver damage and vein lesions are Pyrrolizidine alkaloids. These elements are found to be substances that have a part in the liver cancer disease in humans.

Different origins of natural poison are tiny algae and plankton in oceans or occasionally in lakes that produce chemical compounds that are lethal to humans but not to fish or shellfish that consume these poison manufacturing organisms. When people eat fish or shellfish that contain these toxins, illness can rapidly follow.

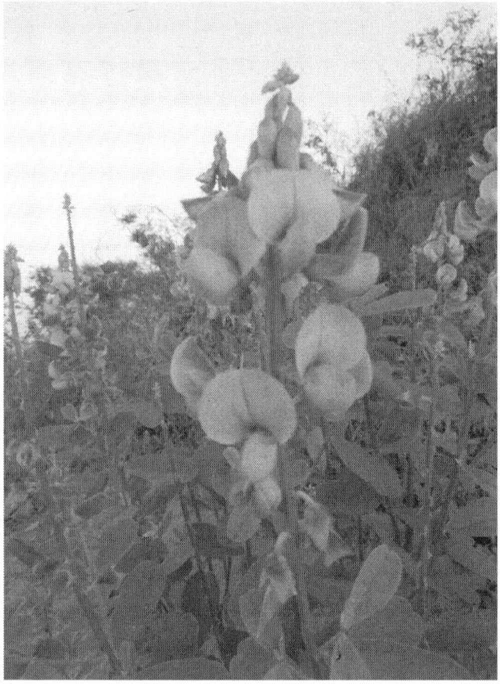

Figure 4.1. Crotalaria.

Source: https://live.staticflickr.com/1844/44741274391_7344ba5a79_b.jpg

Some of the most generally found natural toxins that can pose a risk to our health are given below.

4.2.1. Aquatic Biotoxins

The poison produced by algae in the ocean and freshwater is called algal poison. The poison in algae is produced during flowering in specific naturally occurring algal species. The poison is more likely can be found in Shellfish such as mussels, scallops, and oysters than fish. The poison found in algae can cause diarrhea, vomiting, tingling, paralysis, and other things in humans, other mammals, or fish. The algae poison is inside the shellfish and fish or poison drinking water. They have no palate or odor and are not eradicated by cooking or freezing.

For example, the consumption of fish containing dinoflagellates that manufacture ciguatoxins causes ciguatera fish poisoning. The fish that contain ciguatoxins are barracuda, black grouper, dog snapper, and king mackerel. The Indications of ciguatera poisoning are nausea, vomiting, and neurologic symptoms, such as tingling sensation on fingers and toes. Presently there are no particular drugs available for treatment for ciguatera poisoning (Figure 4.2).

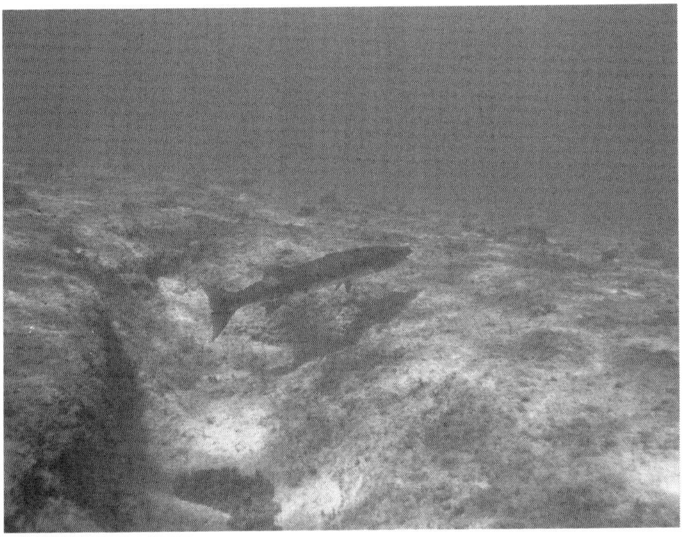

Figure 4.2. Barracuda.

Source: https://cdn12.picryl.com/photo/2016/12/31/barracuda-fish-underwater-travel-vacation-5659fe-1024.jpg

The shellfish that have become poisonous with poison or collection of poison from the consumption of lethal sea plant, especially the contaminated dinoflagellates causes paralytic shellfish poisoning. The shellfish contained are pelecypods, a family of mollusks, including mussels and clams. The dinoflagellates manufacture an intricate blend of poison. One of the main elements that has been recognized as saxitoxin.

The indications of contamination in the human body by shellfish poisoning are stinging and burning in the face, lips, tongue, and finally the whole body, and paresthesia then numbness, general motor imbalance, confusion, and headache. All these indications appear within 30 minutes after consumption. In twelve hours, the difficulty in breathing and then finally death. During the time of blossoming of dinoflagellate that appears red in seawater also known as red tide, though it can be yellowish, brownish, greenish, and bluish. The xanthophyll peridinin is responsible for the red colour (Figure 4.3).

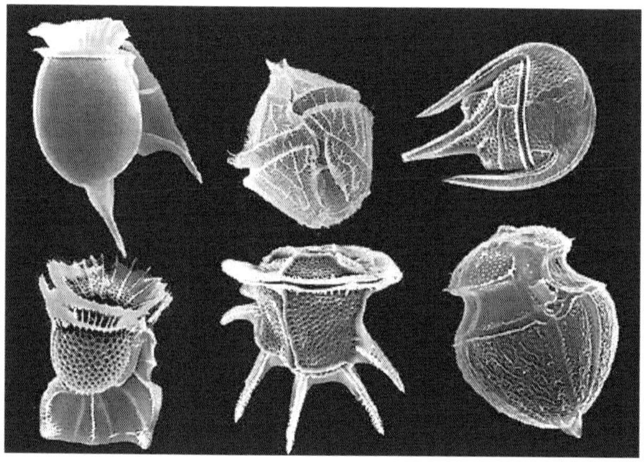

Figure 4.3. Dinoflagellate.

Source: https://live.staticflickr.com/7182/6939384773_3f095e5851.jpg

Normally the high contamination of paralytic shellfish contaminates, intoxication happens that is not existable. This is mainly due to tight guidelines in force in many countries and the alertness in coastal areas of the dangers related to eating shellfish during red tides. Though normal cooking finishes to 70% of the poison and frying in a pan with boiling oil abolishes the remaining, there might be enough poison left in the mollusks to cause serious poisoning.

4.2.2. Cyanogenic Glycosides

The cyanogenic glycosides are phytotoxins are the type of poisonous chemicals manufactured by plants that are found in at minimum 2000 plant varieties, out of which several different types of plants are used as food in some areas of the world. The important foods that have cyanogenic glycosides inside them are cassava, sorghum, stone fruits, bamboo roots, and almonds.

The possible lethality of a cyanogenic plant rests mainly on the possibility that its consumption will manufacture a solution of cyanide that is poisonous to exposed humans. The indications of severe poisoning in humans are fast breathing, low blood pressure, dizziness, headache, stomach pains, vomiting, diarrhea, and mental confusion, cyanosis with jolting and spasms, and lastly coma. The death can happen because cyanide poisoning can happen when the level of cyanide surpasses the limit an individual can detoxify.

4.2.3. Furocoumarins

These types of poison are present in a large number of plants such as parsnips that are closely associated with carrots and parsley, celery roots, citrus plants like lemon, lime, grapefruit, bergamot, and some medicinal plants. Whenever the physical damage to the plant happens then the stress hormones called Furocoumarins are released in response.

In sensitive people, some of these poisons can cause a problem in the intestines. The significant damage to skin under ultraviolet (UV) light under the sun can happen as Furocoumarins are phototoxic. While mainly occurring after dermal exposure, such reactions have also been reported after consumption of large quantities of certain vegetables containing high levels of furocoumarins.

4.2.4. Lectins

A large number of varieties have poison called lectins, and kidney beans contain the largest ever deposit particularly red kidney beans. A small number of fresh beans can start plain stomach ache, vomiting, and diarrhea.

The dry beans if soaked in water for twelve hours before cooking destroys the lectins and then boiled strongly for at least 10 minutes in water. The packaged kidney beans in tin cans have already gone through this process so they can be used without more treatment.

4.2.5. Mycotoxins

The natural poison belonging to another category of poison is called mycotoxins. The word mycotoxin has originated from the Greek word for fungus mykes and the Latin word toxicum meaning poison. Mycotoxins are poisonous chemical products produced by fungi that can grow on crops in the field or after harvest. The eatables that can be infested are cereals, nuts, fruit, and dried fruit, coffee, cocoa, spices, oilseeds, and milk.

Presently there are 300 recognized varieties of mycotoxins of largely different chemical forms and divergent modes of action. These toxins targets are the kidney, liver, or immune system and some are carcinogenic. The general common mycotoxins contain aflatoxins, ochratoxin A, ergot alkaloids, fumonisins, patulin, trichothecenes such as deoxynivalenol which is also known as vomitoxin and zearalenone.

The few types of molds are responsible for the production of naturally occurring poisonous compounds known as mycotoxins. The molds that can

A dangerous level of solanine is found in sprouts. The removal of fruit skin can remove the solanine.

The indications observed in potato poisoning can be due to the combined action of alkaloids as potatoes also contain other glycoalkaloids, mainly chaconine and tomatine, with biological characteristics the same as solanine. Solanine is heat constant and not soluble in water. So poisonous potatoes cannot become less dangerous by cooking. Normally it is accepted that 20 mg solanine/100 g of fresh weight is the upper safety limit.

4.3.8. Biogenic Amines

They are less in weight with organic bases and are a danger to biological activity. Naturally present in animals, plants, and microorganisms.

They are mainly found in fermented foods, vegetables, meats. They are generated by the enzymatic decarboxylation of amino acids by microorganism origin; high concentration in fish and cheese.

4.3.9. Mushroom Toxins

It is produced by the high level of amatoxins in mushrooms. They are recognized as containing amatoxin toxins are the species Amanita bisporigera, A. temifolia, A. ocreata, A. suballiacea, Galerina autumnalis, and Lipiota brunneolilacea.

There are four types of mushroom toxins.

- The nervous contaminants give rise to neurological symptoms such as profuse sweating, hallucinations, depression, spastic colon, excitement, convulsions, and coma.
- The protoplasmic contaminants give rise to widespread destruction of cells, after that there is a condition of organ failure.
- The intestinal contaminants manufacture fast, momentary nausea, stomach cramps, vomiting, and diarrhea.
- The disulfiram-like toxins are normally nonpoisonous and produce no indications. Though, if alcohol is ingested 72 hours after eating them, it can produce vomiting, nausea, headache, flushing, and cardiovascular disturbances.

4.4. MINIMIZING THE HEALTH RISK FROM NATURAL TOXINS

The natural poison can be found in different types of crops and foodstuff. In a normal sustainable, regular intake, the levels of natural poison are always below the danger level for acute and chronic toxicity.

In order to reduce the from natural poison in food, people are advised to:

- Not assume that if something is 'natural' it is automatically safe;
- Discard the bruised, damaged or discolored food, and specially spoiled foods;
- Discard any food that has no odor or taste fresh, or it does not have regular taste; and
- Only eat mushrooms or other wild plants that have been recognized as safe to eat.

4.5. PLANT TOXINS AND PALATABILITY TO HERBIVORES

The connection between the poison in plants and the deliciousness of such plants to plant-eating humans, especially domesticated animals, are extraordinarily intrinsic. As a result, few studies have been done to associate the presence or nonappearance of a specific toxin in a plant with the tolerability of that plant as a food source for mammalian herbivores.

Although, a significant body of knowledge is there as to the particular phytochemicals answerable for the contamination of specific plant varieties, exclusively, which are accountable for either human poisonings or animal poisonings creating main financial losses to milk rearing animals' producers.

4.5.1. Toxins and Their Role in Plants

The plant must regularly fight with other plants for limited resources found in soil. It is regularly in danger from other plants who are occupying their place on the soil from which it extracts nutrients, by microorganisms, by insects, and by both large and small mammalian, avian, or reptilian herbivores. If plants must grow and live, then every plant must draw upon a complex of defences, it can be physical, for example, pricks or leathery leaves, or chemical.

Normally, these measures are for defence, they become active only when the plant is attacked, though in some situations lethal chemicals might

4.7.1. Paralysis Pea

This type of plant doesn't get affected by drought and the hardy grass pea is grown regularly as a safe crop by small farmers in many places around the world like India and Ethiopia. The protein-rich seed has the same toxin, β-ODAP, found in the wild potato that tribals use as their food.

It is safe in a minute amount, especially if it's been soaked in water for a long time. If any human consumes it more than three or four months then it can start a neurological disorder called lathyrism. For example, in 1942 the Jewish prisoners in a camp in Ukraine have first found this disease in their bodies. The officers of the Nazi party supplied prisoners with flour made from grass pea seeds. It was death by bread. The prisoners have become paralyzed in the lower body. Many prisoners were malnourished and physically exhausted.

4.8. CONCLUSION

The natural toxins are producing by plants by using valuable resources from soil, water, and air and use as arms to fight the predators like insects, molds, and various microscopic organisms which are not visible to the naked eyes but are very dangerous for human bodies if we consume them without properly processing them.

The animals consume these plants and then these toxins reach their bodies and then animals' bodies react to these toxins and develop various types of diseases. The marine fishes also develop toxins inside their bodies as the fighting mechanism against predators and to protect them from being hunted. The toxins passed from plants in human bodies with food and then our bodies react to them and develop the disease. The toxins are also beneficial for our bodies as the medical field is researching to make medicines with these toxins.

REFERENCES

1. Canada.ca., (n.d.). Natural Toxins – Canada.ca. [online] Available at: https://www.canada.ca/en/health-canada/services/food-nutrition/food-safety/chemical-contaminants/natural-toxins.html (Accessed on 14 May 2019).
2. Ellen, B. R., (2013). NPR Choice Page. [online] Npr.org. Available at: https://www.npr.org/sections/thesalt/2013/10/01/228221063/when-edible-plants-turn-their-defenses-on-us (Accessed on 14 May 2019).
3. Molyneux, J. R., & Ralphs, H. M., (n.d.). [online] Journals.uair.arizona.edu. Available at: https://journals.uair.arizona.edu/index.php/jrm/article/download/8677/8289 (Accessed on 14 May 2019).
4. Shull, L., & Cheeke, P., (n.d.). Effects of Synthetic and Natural Toxicants on Livestock. [eBook] p. 2. Available at: https://pdfs.semanticscholar.org/9493/08e902c90a710906d9498dec07d9c5beb222.pdf (Accessed on 14 May 2019).
5. Srmuniv.ac.in., (n.d.). [online] Available at: http://www.srmuniv.ac.in/sites/default/files/downloads/food_and_toxicity_natural_toxins.pdf (Accessed on 14 May 2019).
6. Tang, S. P. D., (2007). An Overview of Natural Toxins in Food. [online] Cfs.gov.hk. Available at: https://www.cfs.gov.hk/english/multimedia/multimedia_pub/multimedia_pub_fsf_11_02.html (Accessed on 14 May 2019).
7. WHO.int., (2018). Natural Toxins in Food. [online] Available at: https://www.who.int/news-room/fact-sheets/detail/natural-toxins-in-food (Accessed on 14 May 2019).

Chapter 5

Risks and Benefits of Food Additives

CONTENTS

5.1. INTRODUCTION

Food additives are substances used by food industries to add to their food in minimal quantity during food production in a way to enhance the organoleptic of the food. The primary objective to use food additives is to increase the overall shelf life of food by ensuring product freshness, wholesomeness, and consistency.

It helps in purchasing and producing the food in large quantities without worrying about daily cooking or shopping. It is important to note that food manufacturers must add additives in required quantities or concentrations as per the food safety standards to ensure that it will not result in harming the health of people. Food additive can be defined as any substance used in the process of production, treatment, processing, storage, transportation, or packaging of food.

Food additives are also used to enhance the taste, flavour, or appearance of the food. Some food additives have been used for many decades. For example, preserving food by pickling (preserving with vinegar), salting, as with bacon, and preserving sweets or using sulfur dioxide as in some wines. With the change in the variety of techniques to process food in the mid of 20th century, many new different types of additives have been introduced, both artificial as well as artificial in nature.

According to the United States Food and Drug Administration (FDA, 1993), food additives can be defined as "any substance, the intended use of which results or may reasonably be expected to result, directly or indirectly, in it becoming a component or otherwise affecting the characteristics of any food." in other terms, it can be defined as any substance that is added to the food. In addition, food additives are chemical substances that are intentionally added to the food, either directly or indirectly in limited quantities for purposes of assisting in the processing of foods; preservation of foods; or in improving the texture, flavour, or appearance of foods.

Food additives can be used directly or indirectly. Direct additives can be defined as those additives that are added intentionally to the food during storing, packaging, or processing. If the purpose to add a particular additive is to achieve a certain objective, then it is called a direct additive. For example, the low-calorie sweetener aspartame that is mostly used in puddings, beverages, chewing gum, yogurt, and other food items is called a direct additive because it is added to add flavour to the food.

The type and quantity of direct additives are printed on the packaging of the food in the column of ingredients, while on the other hand; indirect food additives can be defined as those additives that are automatically added to the food during the process of packaging, handling, or storing of food. For example, some colourants such as canthaxanthin (orange), erythrosine (red), and annatto bixin (yellow-orange) help in attracting the consumers towards a particular food, even those they do not provide nutrients to the food.

It is generally seen that these minimal amounts of packaging substances come in contact with the food in some way during the storage of food. A food preservative is a type of food additive whose primary purpose is to protect the food from external environment conditions or of any pathogenic microorganisms such as Bacillus cereus, Clostridia, Staphylococcus aureus, and other microorganisms.

Food preservatives help in preserving the food by reducing the pH level and also stabilizing the redox potential of the food to ensure that microorganisms do not survive in this environment. Food additives are further categorized into two types; natural and synthetic. The natural ones are derived from natural sources such as animals, plants, and minerals, while the synthetic ones are created artificially.

In the present scenario, it is mostly observed that people like food that is ready-made or easy to cook. In these types of foods, preservatives, and additives are mostly used to enhance the flavour and ensure the longevity of the product so that they are not spoiled by bacteria and yeasts. Currently, approximately more than 3000 additives and preservatives are available in the market that is mainly considered as antioxidants and antimicrobial agents.

Some of the food additives and preservatives that are mostly used in preserving and securing food are amino acid compounds, aluminum silicate, sodium nitrate, ammonium carbonates, butylated hydroxytoluene (BHT), monosodium glutamate (MSG), butylated hydroxyanisole (BHA), white sugar, salt, potassium sorbate, potassium bromates, and sodium benzoate. Some artificial colours that are also mostly used in food to make them more attractive to customers are canthaxanthin (orange), erythrosine (red), tartrazine (Azoic yellow), amaranth (Azoic red), and annatto bixin (yellow-orange)

It is important to note that to increase the longevity of the product, adding additives and preservatives is important to enhance food quality, taste, wholesomeness, flavour, and appearance. Food with a great number of water results in the activation of fungi, bacteria, and yeasts within the food, resulting in food spoilage.

The use of additives and preservatives minimize the risk of food spoilage by preventing the growth and development of fungi and bacteria. Additives and preservatives help in maintaining the quality and freshness of the foods. They also maintain palatability and wholesomeness of the food improve or maintain its nutritional value, provide leavening a colour, control appropriate pH, and increasing the flavour of the food.

There are many types of chemicals and compounds that are used during the preparation of food to make it more appealing to customers, enhancing its overall taste, texture, and colour. Food additives are also used in a way to prevent the growth of microorganisms such as bacteria and mold – for the purpose to increase the longevity of the product, which means a longer expiry date, thus improves overall profitability.

However, apart from the few benefits, there are many harmful effects of food additives as it may result in causing an allergic reaction and other health concerns to the people consuming foods having food additives.

5.2. WHAT IS A FOOD ADDITIVE?

Whenever a person looks at the label of any food packaging, the first few ingredients that they read are those that are commonly used in the home such as sugar, flour, and salt, and any person that reads the food label can easily recognize this. However, some of the ingredients that usually appear at the bottom of the list are the ones that most people do not know about.

Some of them are sorbic acid, monoglycerides, and sodium benzoate. They may appear unfamiliar to people when they look at it, and they may think what these are? Why they are present in food? What is the role of these ingredients? Are they safe for consumption? These types of ingredients are food additives.

A food additive is anything that may have a certain impact on food either directly or indirectly or is a component of food. Legally, a food additive is any substance that is added to food during the process of food production, i.e., not on the 'Generally Recognized as Safe' (GRAS) list.

The GRAS list comprises food substances such as sugar, flour, and salt – any ingredient that has been used for a long period of time and does not seem to have any adverse effects on the human body. Thus, food manufacturing companies need to get government approval before adding any type of additive to food. When it comes to food additives, there are different viewpoints of experts, food companies, and governments about how safe they are and what is the safe quantity to use additives in food. Before the approval of the government for any type of food additive, it is vital to do proper studies and research to know how safe it is and what is its impact on the health of humans.

If further research ever shows a food additive to have adverse effects, then the government has the right to remove that additive from the approved list.

5.2.1. Why Are Food Additives Used?

The primary purpose to use food additives by food industries is to make sure that their food lasts longer, is free from bacteria, and the taste and texture of food remain stable and uniform. It is also used to enhance the taste of food and make it more appealing to customers.

It is commonly seen that most of the food that anyone buys from the grocery store is not fresh and present on the shelf of food store for few days, and even weeks and it is possible only by using food additives and preservatives in large quantity. There are many other reasons for food additives being used as well.

Food additives can be used as a preservative, colour, flavour, no-calorie sweetener, nutrient addition, fat replacer, stabilizer, emulsifier, pH control, thickener, anti-caking agent, leavening, humectant (to hold in moisture), enzyme preparation, and dough strengthener.

5.3. RISKS OF FOOD ADDITIVES

Food additives are primarily categorized into many types based on their functions and usability. The most common types of food additives are sweeteners, preservatives, flavourings, colouring agents, stabilizers emulsifiers, thickeners, acidity control agents, texturizers, anti-caking compounds, leavening agents, and humectants that plays an important role in maintaining moisture in the food.

Detailed descriptions of food additives are provided on the label of the food packaging, but their role or primary functions are not provided on the label.

5.3.1. Allergic Reactions

The chances to have an allergic reaction from the food additives exist if the immune system of a person considers it pathogenic or disease-causing.

According to a Turkish study published in a 2012 edition of "Clinical Reviews in Allergy and Immunology," sensitivities or allergic reactions to food additives may be proliferating, especially over the last 20 years.

Furthermore, allergic reactions to food additives are usually mild; skin irritation, intestinal upset, some breathing problems, so they may be greatly under-reported. In addition, according to a study published in the year 2009 in "Current Opinion in Allergy and Clinical Immunology," it was found that allergic reactions from food additives reached 7% and mostly prevails in those people that are more vulnerable to eczema, a type of skin rash.

There are certain harmful chemicals present in food additives such as sulfites, MSG, artificial sweeteners, and food colourings that may cause allergic reactions or asthma.

5.3.2. Links to ADHD

It was observed that attention deficit hyperactivity disorder or ADHD has been increased over the last 20 years, and doctors and researchers are continuously involved in studies to find out the reason for this disease. It can be said that an increase in the disease may be due to improvement in the technique of diagnosis or maybe an increase in the addition of food additives and preservatives that the children consume.

Some earlier research, such as a study published in a 1994 edition of the journal "Annals of Allergy," it was found that there is a direct relationship between the consumption of preservatives and artificial colours and the problem of ADHD.

On the other hand, based on the studies conducted by the Mayo Clinic, it stated that there is no solid proof that food additives cause ADHD, but certain preservatives and food colours may contribute to increasing hyperactive behaviour in some children. Chemicals linked to hyperactivity include red food dye, sodium benzoate, and various yellow food dyes.

5.3.3. Potential Links to Cancer

There are different types and variety of food additives such as saccharin, aspartame, benzoates, and nitrites that may result in causing cancer based on studies conducted on animals as they produce carcinogenic compounds when they are metabolized, according to the Center for Science in the Public Interest. This is one of the controversial topics as many studies contradict each other, but according to FDA, currently, there is no human research that proves this claim that removing any of these chemicals from food, and any metabolites produced from these compounds are of low enough quantity to be harmless.

5.4. THE 12 MOST DANGEROUS FOOD ADDITIVES AND HOW TO AVOID THEM

Whenever you go to a grocery store, have you ever asked questions from yourself that how long these energy bar lasts on the shelf from which you purchase these? (Figure 5.1)

Nutrition Facts	
Serving size	**100 grams**
Amount Per Serving	
Calories	**280**
	% Daily Value*
Total Fat 6g	**8%**
Saturated Fat 0.8g	**4%**
Trans Fat 0g	
Polyunsaturated Fat 3.27g	
Monounsaturated Fat 1.5g	
Cholesterol 0mg	**0%**
Sodium 100mg	**4%**
Total Carbohydrate 10g	**4%**
Dietary Fiber 54g	**193%**
Total Sugars 0g	
Includes 0g Added Sugars	**0%**
Protein 20g	**40%**
Vitamin D 0mcg	0%
Calcium 419mg	30%
Iron 6mg	35%
Potassium 961mg	20%
Magnesium 243mg	60%

*The % Daily Value (DV) tells you how much a nutrient in a serving of food contributes to a daily diet. 2,000 calories a day is used for general nutrition advice.

Figure 5.1. Description of food additives on food packaging.

Source: https://upload.wikimedia.org/wikipedia/commons/b/bc/Wattleseed_Nutrition_Label.png

Food additives and preservatives are important self-defensive tools used by food manufacturing industries to increase the shelf life of the product, protect it from external environmental conditions, and make it more appealing to customers. Food scientists and researchers develop some innovative techniques to make sure food looks and tastes terrific long after it would naturally decompose.

These additives are easily approved because of the policy of the authorities to try them in small quantities, but these are not consumed in small quantity, resulting in harming the health of the person. It is important to note that presently, most of the food found in grocery stores is either pre-packed, genetically modified (GM), or includes chemicals to maintain the taste and freshness. Today, our national food supply is better suited to a nation of plastic mannequins than a nation of real humans.

Marketers are justified in their claim that in fact, these additives help in improving the quality of food by preventing the growth of microorganisms in foods and also lower the cost of the food. However, all these claims are false without any significant proof. No one can deny the fact that food additives impact health significantly. Some of the food additives with their potential danger and ways how to prevent them are discussed below:

5.4.1. BHT (Butylated Hydroxytoluene) and BHA (Butylated Hydroxyanisole)

It is a type of additive that is mostly used in processed foods to prevent oxidation. In 2005, National Toxicology Program listed it as 'reasonably anticipated to be a human carcinogen' and it's used in jet fuels, embalming fluid, rubber petroleum products, and transmission fluid.

BHA is generally added to foodstuffs and oil to prevent spoiling. In various research and studies were undertaken, it was found that these additives may result in contributing to the growth of cancerous tumours in rats.

5.4.2. High Fructose Corn Syrup (HFCS)

It is well known that most of the famous breakfast cereals and pre-packaged treats are loaded with HFCS. It was observed that carbonyl molecules present in HFCS may damage tissue, which results in causing obesity, diabetes, and heart-related disease. It makes the case, even more, worsen when HFCS is made from GM corn and is processed with GM enzymes. The sample of HFCS made with these has also tested positive for mercury.

Proponents of HFCS made a point that if these are eaten in a reasonable quantity, then it will not have a negative impact, but it is not true at all. Here's why. High Fructose Corn Syrup (HFCS) shuts down the brain's ability to discern fullness and increases the desire to eat. HFCS does not cause health issues if eaten in moderate quantity, but practically it is not possible. When a person starts eating food, his capacity to consume food increases. That's why those who drink diet soda gain more weight rather than reducing it.

5.4.3. Soybean Oil

Aside from the fact this is a partitioned food that helps in gaining weight and causes cravings, there is a high probability that the processed food one eats may contain soybean oil that is produced from genetically modified soybeans. It is important to note that currently, most of the soybean crops produced in the United States are GM. It is widely believed that GMOs are not good for the environment, and present studies proved that it is dangerous for the health of humans. With the dangers of GMOs still largely unanticipated, consumers are unwitting guinea pigs.

This is not unlike the times when cigarettes were thought to be safe. No one wanted to believe the corporate manipulation and the biological dangers, but now there are large numbers of addicted people who are dying because they are unable to quit smoking. GM Foods are doing the same thing.

All over the world, there are large numbers of people who are sick and dying but unable to leave food because they become habitual for a particular food. Real foods don't cause cravings. Only the foods that contain additives make the consumer develop the habit to eat that food. Thus, a consumer should always be cautious before eating any type of food. It should always check the label of food before eating it always check for additives and preservatives that are harmful to health.

5.4.4. Propylene Glycol Alginate (E405)

This type of additive is primarily used as a thickener, stabilizer, and emulsifier in many processed foods. Apart from the food companies, it is also used in many industrial components such as airport runway deicers and automotive antifreeze. However, there are so many natural thickeners available that can be used in place of this.

5.4.5. Polysorbate 60

Polysorbates are a group of emulsifiers that are generally used in the pharmaceutical industry and food processing industries.

Food in which polysorbate 60 is mainly used is frozen desserts, imitation cream, baked goods, and frozen desserts to increase the longevity of the product and maintain the taste during the product life.

5.4.6. Enriched Flour

It is well known that people generally prefer the term 'enriched' as the one that is only enhanced with nutrients. However, the enrichment that is used in enriched flour are toxic chemicals such as a metallic form of iron, and the human body cannot absorb this. Naturally, the human body will be faced with the work of cleaning out those heavy metals.

Nowadays, it is generally seen that term enriched is used by marketers actively to sell their products and change the perception of customers. Enriched is misinterpreted by the customer as healthier; in fact, it harms the health of a person.

5.4.7. Olestra

This type of additive is mostly used in potato chips that are free from fat. It mostly does its job by providing chips that are free from calories, fat, and cholesterol, but it may result in causing cancer by binding to fat-soluble vitamins A, D, E, and K. When these types of nutrients aren't being suffocated by olestra, they play an important role in providing vital nutrients that enhance immunity and protect the body from cancer. In the real world, there are no shortcuts.

If it isn't real food, then it's a toxin. It's that simple, and everyone should avoid toxins as much as possible, and if the body comes in contact with toxins by some means, then it should use its preciously scarce resources to rid itself of the poison. And while it's doing that, it can't be doing more important things, like protecting you from the latest flu virus going around.

5.4.8. Propyl Gallate

It is a type of preservative that is mostly used in vegetable oils, meat products, soup mixes, and chewing gum to prevent spoiling. According to certain studies and research, it was found that regular consumption of food containing these may result in causing stomach and colon cancer.

The best way to avoid these problems is to read the label of food packaging before consumption of food. People should not buy industrialized animal products, processed, and food containing preservatives and partitioned oils, and easy to make soup cartons.

These foods might be tasty and save cooking time but are not good for health. By overeating processed foods, people gradually like the taste of these foods and not being able to enjoy the natural tastes of real foods.

Initially, people do not like the taste of real food, but after some time, the human body cleanses itself of all the excite-toxins, and people will heal and regain the taste of real foods again.

5.4.9. Potassium Bromate

It is well known that most people prefer bread in their breakfast, but they are not aware of the fact Potassium bromate is an oxidizing agent that is mostly used in the bread-making process.

This type of additive has carcinogenic effects and is not good for the kidneys. In a study conducted on rats, bread was given to them containing this additive, and it was found that after eating bread for a certain period, they developed kidney tumors and thyroid.

5.4.10. Monosodium Glutamate (MSG)

MSG considers as among the most dangerous additives and is linked to migraines, skin rashes, seizures, nausea, and heart irregularities. It was found that as people become aware of the potential impact of MSG, food manufacturing companies are involved in practices to hide MSG from the label by using interrelated terms such as citric acid, textured soy protein concentrate, maltodextrin, carrageenan, disodium inosinate, disodium guanylate, and modified corn starch.

It is a type of toxin that can break through the blood-brain barrier. This harmful impact from MSG is enough to avoid the product containing MSG.

5.4.11. Aspartame, Acesulfame-K, and Other Artificial Sweeteners

It is generally seen that people to avoid calories intake present in regular sodas drink sodas that are sugar-free or diet versions. As a result, they consumed drinks that are loaded with artificial sweeteners and aspartame. When it is consumed by the person, the human body converts aspartame into formaldehyde, which may result in causing seizures, migraines, vision loss, MS, and Parkinson's disease.

Presently, a new type of artificial sweetener known as Acesulfame-K is mostly used in baked foods and soft drinks. It was found that it may cause cancer and affects the thyroid gland based on the studies conducted on mice. In the end, it is safely assumed that drinks without sugar-free are far better than drinks with artificial sweeteners. However, pure drinking water should be preferred as compared to soft drinks. There simply is no substitute for the clean water our bodies need to flush toxins and satisfy thirst.

5.4.12. Food Colourings

It is important to be aware people that the foods they consume that have different colours such as jellybean are harmful to their health. These artificial colours, mostly attract customers and also enhance the taste of food, but these are not good for health as they don't come from natural food sources.

It is important to note that most of the food colourants such as Yellow #5 are derived from coal tar, which has the risk to cause cancer and can be loaded with up to 10ppm of lead and arsenic.

5.5. SOME OTHER DANGEROUS FOOD ADDITIVES (FIGURE 5.2)

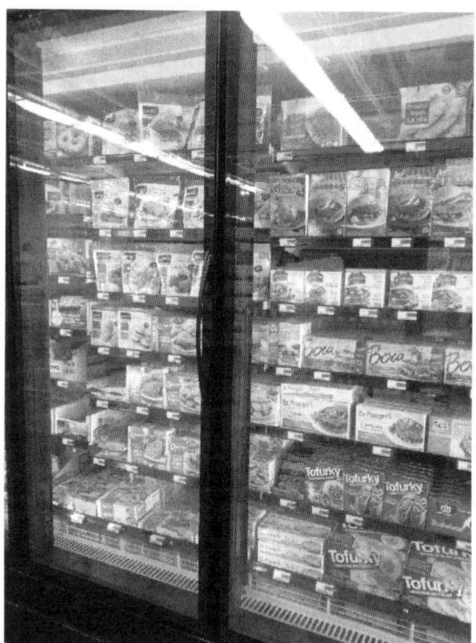

Figure 5.2. Use of additives in processed foods.

Source: https://upload.wikimedia.org/wikipedia/commons/thumb/4/48/Vegan_processed_food%2C_July_2014.jpg/2448px-Vegan_processed_food%2C_July_2014.jpg

5.5.1. Trans Fats

This type of additive is mostly found in processed foods, and it is directly linked to colon cancer, Alzheimer's disease, diabetes, high blood pressure, coronary heart disease, and liver dysfunction. In certain studies, it was found that this may cause infertility in women and also cause obesity problems. The only way to prevent the consumption of trans fat is to avoid processed food completely. Trans Fats are created when heat is applied to oil.

Keep in mind that oil is a partitioned food that does not come in the category of whole food. Whole foods have built-in protections, but once a part is separated from the whole, a problem occurs. Apart from fats present in seeds, nuts, avocados, and good olives, all other whole raw foods contain traces of fat anyway.

But once the fat is collected from these sources and then add high heat, then this is called Trans Fats. Fat is good but when it is in a natural state. Thus, it is recommended that we never consume processed food because the chances of trans fat in these foods are very high.

5.5.2. Chloropropanols

This type of additive is so dangerous that it is even banned in many countries as it is directly linked to different types of cancer. This type of additive is primarily found in sauces that are manufactured in Asian countries. Some of the sauces in which it is found are soy, black bean, and oyster sauces. Remember, not all countries have safety laws in their food supplies. As in Asia, most the countries are developing, so there is no strict regulation for food protection and safety.

It is important to be aware public as well as food-producing countries about its potential hazard and what is the best alternative available to avoid this additive. It was observed that restaurants, mostly used these types of additives as their ultimate goal are only to enhance the taste of food and to engage in cost-cutting measure practices, resulting in compromising the health of their customers. Thus, individual has to protect their health as well as their family. This means adopting a lifestyle less dependent on restaurants.

5.5.3. Sodium Sulfite (E221)

Sodium sulfite is a type of additive that is mostly used during the winemaking process and is also used in some other types of processed food. According to a recently conducted study by the FDA, it was found that one in every hundred people is sensitive to sulfites in food and those that are vulnerable to sulfite may result having headaches, breathing problems, and rashes.

The highest level of danger is that it may even cause death by cardiac arrest. And that's a pretty severe side-effect of enjoying a glass of wine with dinner. Be very careful. Alcohol is not healthy at all, but most people do not believe this fact. Any nourishment that a person gets from a glass of wine can also be available from the raw fruit from which it was made. Avoid Sulfites whenever it is possible.

5.5.4. Sodium Nitrate/Nitrite

This type of additive is mostly used as a preservative, colouring, and flavouring agent for processed meats such as hot dogs, bacon, and others. Its primary role is to prevent the growth of the botulism-causing bacteria, Clostridium botulinum. There are significant dangerous health impacts that are directly linked to this additive. Some of them include lung disease, cancer-causing agents, vomiting, headaches, migraines, respiratory problems, and cardiovascular problems.

There are different types of food alternatives available that are a far better option than an eating hot dog and also provide good nutritional value. In addition, a person should also avoid eating processed meats as their dangerous impact exceeds their benefits. It is also recommended to adopt a healthy lifestyle by eating foods that are free from additives and are not linked to any disease.

5.5.5. Sulphur Dioxide (E220)

This type of additive is mostly found in soft drinks, beer, dried fruit, wine, vinegar, juices, and cordials, and is directly linked to problems such as low blood pressure, bronchial problems, and anaphylactic shock. In addition, this type of additive is strictly prohibited for consumption by children as its effect on children multiplies.

A person should drink natural and fresh juices that are made at home and are free from any preservative and additive. Avoid drinks containing Sulphur-Dioxide as much as possible as long-term exposure to this may have a significant health impact.

5.6. WHAT IS THE DIFFERENCE BETWEEN ARTIFICIAL AND NATURAL FLAVOURS?

In reality, both artificial, as well as natural flavours, are created by flavour chemists. A flavourist generally uses "natural" chemicals at the time of making natural flavourings while on the other hand, "synthetic" chemicals are used to make artificial flavourings. The chemicals that the flavourists used in producing flavours are the same both in artificial and natural flavours.

This is done in a way to ensure that the flavouring agent is tasted as close or as real as the flavour should be. It is usually done by keeping in mind the taste and preferences of consumers. The primary difference between the two flavourings–natural versus artificial–comes from the source of the chemicals.

It is one of the popularly asked questions that why food manufacturers highlighted a key difference between two flavours on the label of the food. This might be because of the habit of customers to simply buy those foods that are advertised with "No Artificial Flavours" or "All-Natural Ingredients."

When it comes down to the bottom line, both natural and artificial flavouring agents are very chemically similar, and food with natural ingredients is typically more costly.

5.7. SUGGESTIONS TO PREVENT OR MINIMIZE POTENTIAL IMPACT FROM FOOD ADDITIVES

5.7.1. Mislabeling and Secret Ingredients

According to the rules and regulations of the FDA, food manufacturing companies are legally bound to list certain substances such as MSG and sulfites on food labels because of their known risks or side effects. However, it is generally seen that most of the manufacturing companies involved in the practices use interrelated terms instead of the original term to mislead consumers.

For example, some of the term mostly used by food manufacturing companies is "spices" or "flavourings" instead of by the specific name. Some of these are secret ingredients they prefer not to reveal to their competitors.

As it is widely believed that MSG can cause nausea and headaches in some people; therefore food companies change it on the food label and listed it as "natural flavour" or "hydrolyzed yeast." Just like this, there are so many terms that are used interchangeably for harmful additives to hide them from consumers as well as from food-regulated agencies.

5.7.2. Danger of Long-Term Exposure

The FDA regulations state that some of the food substances that are hazardous to humans or animals must be used in small quantities as using them in large quantity may have a significant health impact on human's health. They are of the view that these substances are used in such a small quantity that they are not at all can cause any negative impact on the health of humans. However, most of the studies have not looked at the dose-related effects of these additives.

One cannot deny the fact these may have no impact when used in small quantities, but when used for a long time, gradually it could accumulate in the human body and may cause potential health risks to humans. These substances may not be completely excreted and instead stored in small amounts, which over time may be toxic within your organs.

5.7.3. Risk of Additive Effects

A single additive or preservative may be at low risk or may not cause any risk at all, but no one is exposed to just a single or a few chemicals. Together, when these substances are gradually added to the body and interact with other additives already present in the body may result in producing side chemicals that are hazardous to human health.

In addition, processed food that humans mostly consume not only contains a single additive, but there also are multiple and different varieties of food additives available in a single food, and whose potential side effect in combination is even unknown to researchers as there is no study based on this category. Given this, it is may not be possible to tell in the long which specific food substance caused a health problem. Also, the lower the grade of food, the higher the chances that it contains so many additives to try to enhance it and make it more appealing.

5.7.4. Danger from Indirect Substances

Many chemicals can come in contact with processed food without being intentionally added by the food manufacturer during the processing and refining of foods.

This includes:

- Pesticides that are used by farmers during growing plant foods;
- Hormones, antibiotics, and metals, and other residues from the food animal industry;
- Carbon monoxide or carbon dioxide that is mostly used in food packaging to replace oxygen to preserve color;
- Substances that get into foods from plastic, Styrofoam, or another packaging.
- There is also danger from food additives and preservatives that enter the water supply from discarded foods or during the manufacturing process.

5.7.5. Read Food Labels

It is widely known that some of the people are involved in practices of producing their food, preservatives, and additives play an important in preventing spoilage from the air, moisture, microorganisms, and natural aging of foods and extend shelf life. In addition, added nutrients such as folic acid are also helpful for human health. However, due to too many large categories and different varieties of synthetic and natural substances are available, it is unknown which has the potential benefits and which is hazardous to human health.

Thus, as there is not enough information available concerning health risks of many of these substances, it is suggested to eat a healthy diet, free from preservatives and additives, preferably locally grown, and limit convenience foods. However, it is not possible to avoid these kinds of foods entirely, but whenever a person purchases a food, it is important to read the bottom of food labels and acquire complete information about what a person is eating. Be aware of additives disguised under different names and research any that you don't recognize.

5.8. VARIOUS BENEFITS OF FOOD ADDITIVES

It is mostly experienced by every individual that whenever they look at a food label, there is a large list printed on it and some include frightening names such as alpha-tocopherol, ascorbic acid, and beta-carotene that the consumer is unaware of it. Most of the ingredients do not look familiar, but they are. There are other names for some essential minerals and vitamins that the consumer should consume regularly in their life. Alpha-tocopherol refers to vitamin E, ascorbic acid to vitamin C, and beta-carotene to vitamin A.

Some of the benefits of food additives are discussed below:

5.8.1. Increase Shelf Life

It is important to note that those foods that are infected with microorganisms may cause food poisoning or other health problems. Additives play an important role in keeping the food fresh and also prevented it from spoilage. It plays a major role in preventing the growth of bacteria and viruses on food (Figure 5.3).

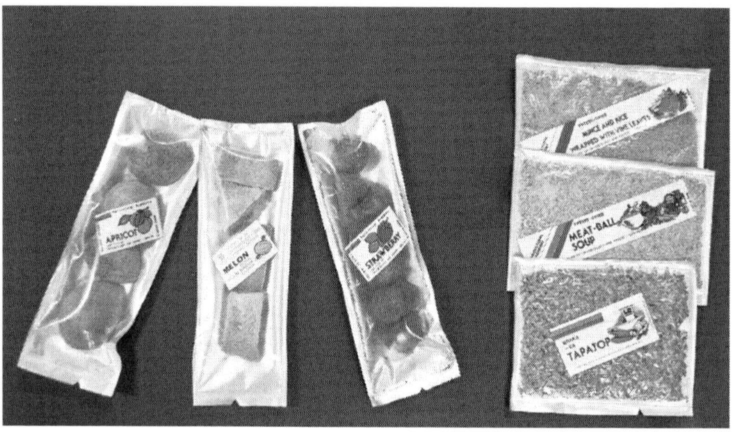

Figure 5.3. Food additives help in increasing shelf life of food products.

Source: https://upload.wikimedia.org/wikipedia/commons/4/45/Bulgarian_space_food.jpg

Salt and other natural additives are commonly used in foods to increase their shelf life. In addition, there is no negative impact of using natural additives. Thus, additives help in maintaining the quality of food for a longer period.

5.8.2. Enhance Flavour

It is well known that certain activities involved in the process of food production such as dehydrating, canning, or freezing to increase the shelf life may alter the flavour of the food. Thus, food manufacturing companies used certain additives such as flavour enhancers, acids, or sweeteners that make the taste of the food better. For instance, the added salt in chips and other fried food leaves you craving for more.

5.8.3. Increase Nutrients with Fortification

During the process of food production, certain minerals and vitamins may get lost. Some foods such as corn flakes are fortified with vitamins, minerals, or fiber for added nutrition.

Preserving food through additives helps in keeping the food for a longer period without losing essential nutrients; thus, it increases the convenience of storing. In addition, it is also helpful in maintaining as well as improving the nutritional value of food. Food enhanced with additives may provide nutrition to a person who does not consume a balanced diet.

5.8.4. Preserve Texture and Appearance

The manufacturing process of food may result in altering the texture as well as the flavour of food, thus making it unpleasant. Natural and artificial flavouring substances, sweeteners, and spices are used in food with the main purpose of preserving the food's texture and appearance.

Emulsifiers and stabilizers help in maintaining the consistency of foods. For instance, a leavening agent added to bakery products helps make them rise.

5.8.5. Safe and More Nutritious Food

Nutritional additives help in enhancing the overall value of food products. In addition, the use of additives and preservatives also increases the safety of food by maintaining its quality and increase its shelf life. The use of antioxidants helps in preventing the development of rancidity and is concerned with maintaining the nutritional value of vitamins and lipids (Figure 5.4).

While antimicrobial agents play an important role in preventing microbial growth in food products. Some of the nutritional additives such as minerals and vitamins are used in many types of food products to add value to the food and prevent nutritional deficiencies if any.

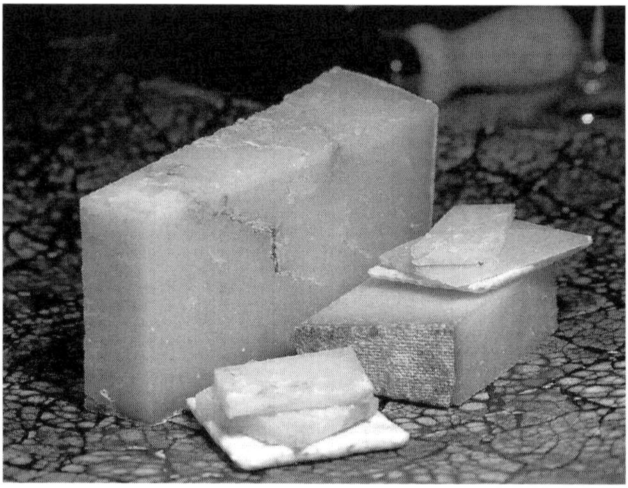

Figure 5.4. Food additives help in preventing food from spoilage.

Source: https://upload.wikimedia.org/wikipedia/commons/2/2e/Montgomerys_cheddar_cheese.jpg

5.8.6. Greater Choice of Foods

Today, customers have a great choice of food products. Due to the use of different types and categories of food additives, there is a different variety of food products available in the market. One of the benefits of food additives is that consumers may even consume food products that are not even seasonal; thus, it gives consumers wide choice to select among different categories of food.

In addition, by the use of additives, there is a significant development in low-calorie and functional foods in the market. Various alternatives of food such as soy meat products and margarine are also gaining importance. Additives play an important role in maintaining the texture, flavour, and nutritional value of food products. According to some studies and researches, it was found that antioxidants help in increasing the shelf life of food products by up to 200%.

Currently, there is a variety of food snacks item available in the market only because of the use of different flavours and colours.

It also provides different options to diet-conscious people as it enables them to consume low-calorie food items. The use of non-nutritive sweeteners such as Aspartame and Cyclamate is increasing instead of sucrose. Stabilizers and emulsifiers are also aiding in the reduction of lipid contents in food products. Functional foods and the nutraceutical industry are also emerging.

5.8.7. Low-Priced Food

According to the marketers of food manufacturing companies, if they completely remove the use of additives during the process of food production, there will be a surge in the prices of their food. For example, if additives are removed from margarine, then consumers will have to buy its alternative that is high in price, i.e., butter.

The safety and shelf life of the product will be reduced if we remove additives from food items, resulting in increased cost of producing food and thus retail prices of food. While on the other hand, advanced packaging material and increased refrigeration will help in reducing the cost of food products. Food can be produced and sold without additives, but the addition of flavours and colours helps in providing a variety of food products, to customers, at a reasonable cost.

5.8.8. Mass Production

Additives play an important role to produce food on a large scale as it helps in increasing the life of food products, so producers do not need to aware about selling the food in minimum time. They can produce food on a large scale to get economies of scale and sell it when the demand arises.

Apart from the producers of food products, suppliers also don't have to worry about spoilt products and food poisoning.

5.8.9. Reduce Foodborne Diseases

The primary role of using food additives is to prevent or reduce foodborne diseases. It also helps in countering the growth of micro-bacteria and any virus caused by decaying food. It keeps the food safe during its entire life cycle.

Some of the diseases are so hazardous that it may even cause death of person, thus different type of additives is used following the nature of the food in a way to successfully fight from these diseases.

5.8.10. Prevent Build-Up of Fat

Antioxidants that are used in foods in combination with unsaturated fats help in preventing the build-up of fatty deposits around the arteries. It allows the human to consume the food without worrying about the quantity that they consumed because it does not add fat into the body. Thus, it makes the human body healthy.

5.8.11. Reduce Premature Birth

The folic acid supplement is an important source for women as it helps in preventing premature birth and malformation in early pregnancy stages.

5.8.12. Promote the Development of Food Industries

It is generally seen that within the past few years as the introduction and usage of different types of food additives, there has been rapid growth and development in food industries. It enables food manufacturers to produce different varieties and categories of the product, thus give tough competition to their competitors.

Furthermore, it also allows them to reduce their cost of production and use higher profits in the expansion and diversification of their companies. Also, the use of additives enables food companies to provide high nutrition food with good taste and appearance at reasonable prices, thus increasing the goodwill of the company.

5.9. DIFFERENT TYPES OF NATURAL AND DERIVED FOOD ADDITIVES

5.9.1. Emulsifiers and Stabilizers

Emulsifiers play an important role in combining substances with similar properties, which means substances that do not mix well together, such as water and oil.

While on the other hand, stabilizers are concerned with ensuring that these substances will not separate after mixing. Some of the food items in which stabilizers and emulsifiers are used are homogenized milk and ice cream.

5.9.2. Antioxidants

It is well known that chemicals that are present in food when coming in contact with oxygen change their original taste and colour. It makes the food go stale, and the oils and fats go rancid. Thus, the primary purpose to use antioxidants is to ensure that the food preserves its original colour and taste, making it the most vital additive to increase the longevity of food.

5.9.3. Salt

Salt is one of the most important food preservatives aimed at preserving fish and meat. Salt dehydrates food and keeps it dry, resulting in preventing the growth of bacteria, yeast, and mold. Salt is a natural food additive, and it is completely safe to consume salt-cured food, and it also lasts years if it is stored under proper conditions, away from direct sunlight and water.

5.9.4. Sugar

Just like salt, sugar also removes moisture from food and makes food acidic. It maintains an environment in food that is not suitable for the survival and growth of bacteria and for other microbes that decompose food. It is a natural food additive that is free from any side effects and makes food safe and secure.

5.9.5. Vinegar

Vinegar is one of the most widely used food additives that has been used by food manufacturing companies for many decades. It contains 5% acetic acid and kills bacteria and other microorganisms. It also gives a sharp flavour to food with its sour taste. It is a natural food additive and is commonly used in homes to prevent food from bacteria.

5.9.6. Anti-Caking Agents

Anti-caking agents such as sodium bicarbonate prevent the food from clumping or sticking together. It is usually added to powdered milk. It is usually seen that certain foods when coming in contact with air stick together because it absorbs moisture in it, thus anti-caking agents play an important role in tackling this problem.

5.10. FUTURE OF NATURAL FOOD ADDITIVES IN COLOURS AND FAT REPLACERS

5.10.1. Packaged Facts

In recent years, it has been observed that sales of foods containing additives and preservatives are declining, while at the same time foods claiming to

Thus, it becomes the responsibility of consumers to carefully read labels before purchasing any kind of foods and should also be aware of different types of popular additives and their health and benefits. Also, consumers should always prefer food that contains natural additives and if possible, then purchase only those foods that do not contain any type of food additive. Furthermore, they should be also aware of the disease that may cause by long-term exposure to food additives.

REFERENCES

1. Faithful palate, (2019). The 17 Most Dangerous Food Additives and How to Avoid Them – Faithful Palate. [online] Available at: https://www.faithfulpalate.com/the-17-most-dangerous-food-additives-and-how-to-avoid-them/ (Accessed on 14 May 2019).
2. Food additives (2019). Natural vs. Artificial. [online] Available at: https://kimberlyjchong.wordpress.com/natural-vs-artificial/ (Accessed on 14 May 2019).
3. foodmanufacture.co.uk., (2019). Demand for Natural Additives Drives Growth. [online] Available at: https://www.foodmanufacture.co.uk/Article/2011/09/16/Demand-for-natural-additives-drives-growth (Accessed on 14 May 2019).
4. foodnavigator-usa.com, (2019). Future of Natural Food Additives in Colours and Fat Replacers: Packaged Facts. [online] Available at: https://www.foodnavigator-usa.com/Article/2013/10/29/Future-of-natural-food-additives-in-colours-fat-replacers (Accessed on 14 May 2019).
5. Foodscintech.blogspot.com., (2019). Benefits of Food Additives. [online] Available at: http://foodscintech.blogspot.com/2014/10/benefits-of-food-additives.html (Accessed on 14 May 2019).
6. Greenliving.lovetoknow.com., (2019). [online] Available at: https://greenliving.lovetoknow.com/dangers-food-additives-preservatives (Accessed on 14 May 2019).
7. Healthline, (2019). 12 Common Food Additives — Should You Avoid Them? [online] Available at: https://www.healthline.com/nutrition/common-food-additives#section1 (Accessed on 14 May 2019).
8. Healthyeating.sfgate.com., (2019). The Disadvantages of Food Additives. [online] Available at: https://healthyeating.sfgate.com/disadvantages-food-additives-9213.html (Accessed on 14 May 2019).
9. Mercola.com., (2019). Food Additives Are More Hazardous in Combination. [online] Available at: https://articles.mercola.com/sites/articles/archive/2015/06/10/hazardous-food-additives.aspx (Accessed on 14 May 2019).
10. Pros a Cons., (2019). Pros and Cons of Food Additives – Pros and Cons. [online] Available at: https://www.prosancons.com/food/pros-and-cons-of-food-additives/ (Accessed on 14 May 2019).

11. Shaikh, F., (2019). Some Amazing Advantages of Adding Food Additives to Your Food. [online] Foods for better health. Available at: https://www.foodsforbetterhealth.com/advantages-of-food-additives-34825 (Accessed on 14 May 2019).
12. Study.com., (2019). Food Additives: Definition, Examples & Uses – Video & Lesson Transcript | Study.com. [online] Available at: https://study.com/academy/lesson/food-additives-definition-examples-uses.html (Accessed on 14 May 2019).
13. Verytweet, (2019). Advantages of Food Additives and Their Side Effects – VERYTWEET. [online] Available at: http://www.verytweet.com/2017/05/21/advantages-of-food-additives-and-their-side-effects/ (Accessed on 14 May 2019).

Chapter 6

Clinical Evaluation of Food Additives

CONTENTS

6.1. INTRODUCTION

Food additives are mainly defined as the substances that are added to specific food items to sustain or enhance the taste, safety, texture, appearance, or freshness of food. Some of the food additives have been in use for preservation for over centuries; for example, salt, sugar, or sulphur dioxide in meats, marmalade, and wine, respectively.

Several of the food additives have been developed over time to meet the requirements of food production have been developed over time to meet the requirements of food production, as preparing food on a big scale is very different from making at home on a small scale.

Additives are majorly required to assure processed food remains safe and in a good condition all over its journey from the industrial kitchens or factories, during the transportation to shops and warehouses, and eventually to consumers.

The use of food additives is justified only when their application has a technological requirement, does not necessarily mislead the consumers, and generally serves a well-defined technological function of preserving the nutritional quality of the food as well as enhancing the stability of food.

Food additives can be easily obtained from plants, animals, or minerals, or they can be synthetic. They are intentionally added to the food products to perform specific technological purposes that consumers generally take for granted.

There is a huge amount of food additives that are used in various food items, all of which are designed to do a particular job in making the food safe or attractive. World Health Organization (WHO), together with the Food and Agricultural Organization (FAO), categorizes food additives into three major kinds based upon their function.

A major aim in the clinical testing of food additives is to evaluate the safety aspects that cannot be adequately addressed by non-human studies or by existing data on the exposure of the population.

As segments of the increased number of populations may be exposed to huge quantities of additives for a long time, conventional methods of assessing the safety of these substances may not be sufficient. Testing or evaluating these substances in animals at doses that significantly amplify their projected human exposures may not be possible.

For these substances, human clinical studies may provide supplementary confidence in the safety of the food additive. A food additive usually will be considered appropriate for the clinical testing if the substance is not likely to produce effective toxic cffccts at the level to which the subjects of the clinical study will be exposed.

Usually, this is determined from the outcomes of the studies of toxicity in animals or by evaluating the current data on the population exposure. Although, in cases where the kind of toxic response linked with the consumption of food additive by the experimental animals is judged to be harsh, disclosure of various subjects in the clinical studies of the food additive may require to be notably below the level found to produce no harmful effects in a specific species.

Different from the patients involving in the clinical trials of new drugs, no health benefits are estimated for numerous test subjects in the clinical studies of food additives. Hence, the nature, as well as weight of evidence needed to establish the safety of food products for humans before clinical studies can start, may vary from that needed to support the testing under proper guidelines for the investigation of new drugs.

The clinical studies of food additives will mainly focus on signifying safety: for instance, the safety of an additive that may obstruct the absorption of nutrients, whose status is not certain in the population, may require to be assessed in a clinical study.

6.2. GENERAL CONSIDERATIONS FOR CLINICAL STUDIES OF FOOD ADDITIVES

The major principles for the conduction of clinical trials are comprised in the 8 May, Federal Register: "Statement concerning adequate and well-controlled clinical investigations." This section describes the guidelines that are used to recognize general considerations that are must for the clinical studies of food additives.

Each of the considerations must be addressed explicitly in the protocol of the clinical study. Before conducting a costly as well as a time-consuming clinical trial as a part of the safety evaluation of a food additive, the investigator requires to prepare a defensible rationale for the conduction of human clinical trials and a clear set of aims and objectives.

Adequate and satisfactory preclinical investigations must have been completed, including the tests of toxicity in animals. The outcomes of these tests must create that there is no expected toxicity to the human at doses to be used in the clinical trials. A clear and concise depiction of the design of investigator of the clinical study. Before the commencement of the clinical trial, the investigator must consider different ways in which the quality control of the trial will be documented. Proper documentation of the quality control will make the review of clinical trials easy.

FDA suggests that the investigators use statistical knowledge in the planning, framing, implementation, and analysis of the pre-clinical and clinical trial. Such kind of expertise will help to assure that the planned trial will provide the required information while decreasing the number of subjects and will empower the validity of safety estimates obtained from the trials.

6.3. PRINCIPLES OF SAFETY EVALUATION

Food is known to be a very common source of toxicant exposure to human beings. A large number of naturally occurring toxic contaminants get into the food. The most threatening products are mold growth, which is known as mycotoxins. Mycotoxins generally include carcinogenic aflatoxins.

Whereas, more than 2500 chemical substances supplement in the foods to impart or modify the flavour, texture, and colour of food, to enrich or increase the value of food, or to decrease the cost. In addition to that, approximately 12,000 substances are utilized in such a way that these substances enter into the food supply unintentionally.

A food additive is a regulatory term that comprises a functional component that is normally not consumed as food itself. This component is added intentionally to the food to supplement its processing or to enhance the colour, aroma, taste, texture, consistency, or shelf life.

Additives are not regarded as nutritional substance, even if they contain a nutritive value. The overall method of safety evaluation of the food additives remains organized around four fundamental principles. First is that the investigator assumes that few of the toxicological information is required for every food additive (Figure 6.2).

Second is that the amount of safety data needed for a specific food additive is mainly ordered by the level of concern (LO). Third is that the LO is based on the magnitude of the latent human intake of a food additive and its molecular structure: exposure data, if present, carrying greater weight than the structure alert.

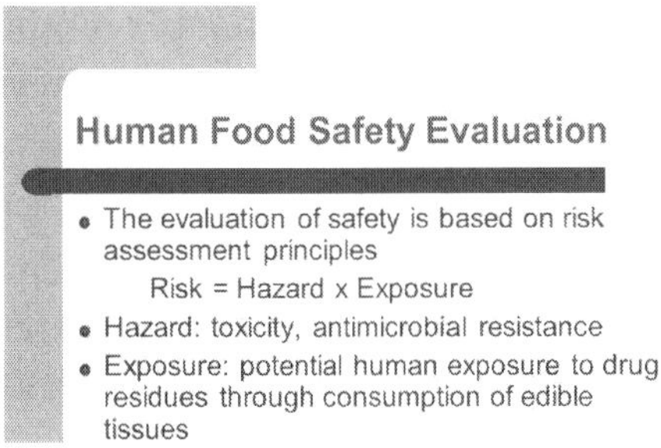

Figure 6.2. Food safety evaluation.

Source: https://slideplayer.com/slide/4607135/

The fourth basic principle is that the initial assessment of testing requirements can be easily adjusted when the data recommend that an effective or unexpected harmful effect is found to be linked with the intake of a specific additive.

The outcomes from the toxicological trials are then used to calculate the ADI (Acceptable Daily Intake) which is contrasted to the EDI (Estimated Daily Intake). If the EDI is less than ADI, the additive is considered to be safe under the current conditions of use or intake.

6.4. FOOD ADDITIVES: AN ETHICAL EVALUATION

A huge amount of different chemicals is supplemented with the processed food items. The great majority of the additives raise some issues in the context of health, but their use is fairly problematic for a significant number.

According to Millstone and Lang, several doubts have been raised related to 200 food additives approximately, which for certain consumers have been declared to cause allergic reactions or acute intolerance, or to extensively increase the risks of serious long-term effects, such as cancer.

A European Community (EC) legislation defined a food additive as 'any substance not normally consumed as a food in itself … the intentional addition of which to food for a technological purpose results in it or its by-products becoming directly or indirectly a component of such foods.'

6.4.1. Ethical Prisms and Principles

Almost any public concern can be observed through a variety of metaphorical prisms, which despite some overlap providing different perspectives and

6.4.3. The Risks of Harm to Consumers

Food additives have been claimed mainly responsible for a great number of disease conditions (it does not include those diseases that are caused due to extreme consumption of fast food). However, some of the assumed associations are perhaps ill-founded, there appears to be strong prima facie evidence for assuring claims.

Numerous groups of public interest have drawn up the lists of food additives, which they consider must be treated with caution or completely avoided mainly by sensitive people. A prominent example is the Center for Science in the Public Interest, whose directors comprise a former FDA commissioner. Theoretically, safety evaluations of food additives might be based on two kinds of evidence, viz. results of toxicological tests and the epidemiological data. In practice, due to the complexity of the diet, lifestyles, and genetic predispositions of people, it is quite possible to derive significant data on the risks of having food additives from epidemiological studies. Exceptions to this generalization prove the rule. For instance, severe harmful reactions to foods known to have certain components may be potentially suggestive of the causal links (as in the quick onset of asthma attacks or various other allergic reactions to certain colourants).

Some severe reactions recommend an allergic response, while others may enforce tolerance. Current estimates are that the allergies caused by food additives affect 3–7% of young children and around 2% of adults in the European nations. Some examples of alleged reactions are given in Table 6.1.

Table 6.1. Alleged Acute Adverse Reactions to Consumption of Certain Food Additives

Organ/System	Examples
Heart	Palpitations; arrhythmias
Digestive	Abdominal pain; nausea; vomiting; colic; flatulence; diarrhoea
Skin	Urticaria; angioedema; pruritus; eczema; rashes
Respiratory	Asthma; coughing; wheezing; rhinitis
Nervous System	Behaviour/mood changes; ADHD; migraine; numbness
Musculoskeletal	Muscle/joint aches; fatigue; weakness

Source: https://academic.oup.com/bmb/article/99/1/7/297198

6.5. THE VALIDITY OF SAFETY EVALUATIONS AND THEIR EFFECTS ON TEST ANIMALS

In the year 1959, William Russell and Rex Burch published the book entitled Principles of Humane Experimental Technique (Russell and Burch, 1959), in which they recommended the "3Rs concept" (refinement, reduction, and replacement) for the humane treatment of the experimental animals.

The 3Rs concept was not identified for around two decades, until the public, as well as scientific communities, became mainly concerned regarding the use of animals in evaluation testing for regulatory and various other purposes.

In regulatory toxicology, animal tests are utilized in the assessment of hazards to recognize the toxicological properties of various chemicals to which people are exposed when these chemicals are used in a specific food item for any specific purpose.

At present, the regulatory safety testing of the drugs and various other chemicals must be done in standardized animal tests. This will initially protect the workers during the production of numerous chemical products, and then it will protect the consumer as well as the environment.

The contact of laboratory animals to different risky chemicals may eventually lead to extensive pain and sometimes even death. To decrease the pain of the laboratory testing animals, the concept of 3Rs has been successfully applied.

At the international level, the harmonization of test guidelines has effectively decreased the testing of animals. It is much tougher to replace a particular animal test applied in regulatory toxicology without decreasing the safety of chemicals.

6.5.1. Reducing the Animal Numbers in Regulatory Testing by International Harmonization of Test Guidelines

From the middle of the 1960s, testing of toxicity has been empirically developed in various laboratories all over the globe. For a particular field of toxicology (such as skin and eye irritation), the standard procedures have varied between different nations (species, regimen of treatment, number of animals per treatment group).

Differences have also been present in the way the information is obtained from the studies of animals has been applied for various regulatory purposes. Current tests of animal safety that should be conducted for various regulatory purposes during the chemical toxicity testing:

- Acute systemic toxicity (oral, dermal, inhalation);
- Carcinogenicity;
- Chronic toxicity;
- Dermal penetration;
- Eye irritation and corrosion;
- Genotoxicity;
- Neurotoxicity;
- Reproductive toxicology;
- Skin irritation and corrosion;
- Skin sensitization;
- Subacute toxicity;
- Subchronic toxicity;
- Teratology and embryotoxicity;
- Toxic kinetics.

6.5.2. Harmonization of the OECD Guidelines for the Testing of Chemicals

The OECD Test Guidelines cover the four major sections:

- Section 1: Physicochemical properties, comprising 20 methods;
- Section 2: Effects on biotic systems, comprising 14 methods;
- Section 3: Degradation and accumulation, comprising 14 methods; and
- Section 4: Health effects, comprising 28 methods on local and systemic toxicity and 15 methods in genetic toxicology.

Differences in the national, as well as international guidelines, are not acceptable from the animal and scientific welfare points of view for economic reasons as repeated or unnecessary testing places imparts burden on the companies working at the international level as well as on the consumer who must give a high price for the final products comprising the tested chemicals.

As a result, industries have persisted in the harmonization of guidelines for chemical testing for various economic reasons. A hurdle to harmonization of test guidelines has been enmity in few nations against the test procedures that are developed abroad.

Alternatively, it is the "NIH did not invent here syndrome," which is still used to keep a marked position. Although, for various economic reasons, companies needed to provide test data to the regulators have used the flexibility and common sense to encourage national as well as international regulatory agencies that harmonization of test guidelines is the only way forward in a global economy.

In the year 1982, the OECD was the first international organization who agreed on the harmonized guidelines for chemical testing. Most significantly, this agreement comprised mutual acceptance of the data produced in the member nations of OECD in studies done as per the guidelines for the chemical testing.

Since then, the same kind of approach has been utilized for the safety as well as efficacy testing of drugs by the International Conference on Harmonization (ICH), which represents the three key economic regions (Europe, Japan, and the United States).

Since the year 1990, the ICH has accepted the harmonized guidelines for the efficacy as well as safety testing of drugs and medicines, including animal tests. The harmonization of test guidelines has led to a considerable reduction of testing in animals in that regulatory agencies over the globe are now accepting the outcomes of tests conducted as per the ICH guidelines.

This reveals that in addition to the drugs, pesticide test and industrial chemical test guidelines have been internationally harmonized for biological and hormones by the pharmacopeias and vaccines by the WHO.

To date, the harmonization of universal test guidelines for safety and toxicity testing has been a successful approach for decreasing animal testing for regulatory purposes.

6.6. SPECIFIC FOOD ADDITIVES

6.6.1. Acidified Sodium Chlorite

Acidified Sodium Chlorite has antimicrobial properties and is intended for use initially as a dipping or spray solution for meats, poultry, fruits, vegetables, and seafood. It is also utilized in the poultry chilling water. Acidified Sodium Chlorite is produced by the addition of a food-grade acid (e.g., citric acid, hydrochloric acid, malic acid, phosphoric acid, or sodium

Then the enzyme is formulated with sodium benzoate, potassium sorbate, and glycerol. The activity of Asparaginase is determined by calculating the rate of hydrolysis of L-asparagine to L-aspartic acid and ammonia. Subsequently, ammonia reacts with α-ketoglutarate to form L-glutamic acid.

The reaction is mainly catalyzed in the presence of NADH by glutamate dehydrogenase. NADH is oxidized to NAD+ with an associated loss of absorbance measured at 340 nm. The activity of asparaginase is measured as a rate of consumption of NADH under standard conditions.

The asparaginase activity is expressed in ASNU activity units. One ASNU is equal to the amount of asparaginase that produces one micromole of ammonia per minute under standard conditions.

6.6.3. Carrageenan and Processed Eucheuma Seaweed

Carrageenan is a substance that has hydrocolloid properties due to the presence of sulfated polyglycans an average molecular mass above 100 kDa. It is generally derived from seaweeds of the Rhodophyceae class.

It does not have any nutritional value, but due to its emulsifying, gelling, and thickening properties, it is used in the preparation of food. Three major kinds of carrageenan are commercially used, which are known as iota, kappa, and lambda carrageenans in the food industry.

These names do not exactly reflect classic chemical structures. They only reflect the general differences in the composition and level of sulfation at particular locations in the polymer. Processed Eucheuma seaweed is derived from either E. cottonii (kappa-carrageenan) or E. spinosum (lambda-carrageenan), also Rhodophyceae.

Carrageenan is obtained by the extraction of seaweed into water or any aqueous dilute alkali. It may be recovered by the precipitation of alcohol, by drum drying, or by precipitation in aqueous potassium chloride and consequent freezing.

The production of processed Eucheuma seaweed comprises the soaking of the cleaned seaweed in alkali for a very short time at an elevated temperature. Then, the treated material is washed thoroughly with the water to remove residual salts and then washed with alcohol, dried, and milled to a powder.

For carrageenan as well as processed Eucheuma seaweed, the alcohols that can be utilized during the process of purification are limited to ethanol, isopropanol, and methanol. Articles of commerce may consist of sugars for standardization, salts to get specific gelling or thickening features, or emulsifiers carried over from drum drying processes.

In a recent study with a classical initiation-promotion protocol, carrageenan at up to 5% in the diet did not encourage colon carcinogenesis in rats commenced by dimethylhydrazine. However, the dietary concentrations of carrageenan that were used in the two studies showed that carrageenan increased colon carcinogenesis in rats much higher and that carrageenan was administered before, during, and after the carcinogens.

Improved carcinogenicity under these situations or conditions may result from the altered toxicokinetics or biotransformation of the carcinogen. Thus, the mechanism of the improvement of colon carcinogenesis in these studies remained unsolved.

Sustained feeding of very high doses of carrageenan formed a global proliferative response, calculated as enhanced activity of thymidine kinase, in the mucosal tissue of the colon of male rats. This effect may play a chief role in the practical improvement of the tumorigenicity of known colon carcinogens by high dietary concentrations of carrageenan.

Although, a proliferative effect of the carrageenan on the mucosa of the colon was observed only with a dietary concentration of carrageenan at 2.6% or higher. Hence, no effect was observed with 1.5% carrageenan in the diet, consequent to 750 mg/kg of body weight per day.

This level deeply surpassed the projected human consumption of processed Eucheuma seaweed or carrageenan of 30–50 mg/person per day from their utilization as a food additive.

6.6.4. Cyclotetraglucose and Cyclotetraglucose Syrup

Cyclotetraglucose is a non-reducing cyclic tetrasaccharide which is consists of four D-glucopyranosyl residues connected by alternating α (1→3) and α (1→6) glucosidic bond. On the other hand, cyclotetraglucose syrup is a mixture of mainly cyclotetraglucose with branched cyclotetraglucose, mono-, and disaccharides, and linear branched or not branched oligosaccharides.

They are mainly formed by the hydrolyzed food-grade starch by the activities of a combination of 6-α-glucosyltransferase (6-GT) and α-isomaltosyltransferase (IMT) that are derived from Sporosarcina globispora and Cyclodextrin glucosyltransferase that is derived from Bacillus stearothermophilus from liquefied food-grade starch as the beginning material by the joint actions of 6-GT and IMT, both isolated from Sporosarcina globispora. Crystalline cyclotetraglucose and cyclotetraglucose syrup are separately produced based on the given steps. Cyclotetraglucose syrup is a mixture of cyclotetraglucose with branched cyclotetraglucose, mono-, and disaccharides, and linear branched or not branched oligosaccharides. The product mainly includes 30–40% of cyclotetraglucose on a dry matter basis.

Crystalline cyclotetraglucose and its aqueous solutions are tasteless as well as odourless. A very small amount of sweetness may be perceived. The amount is so small that it is of no practical relevance. On the other hand, cyclotetraglucose syrup is a little sweet because of coexistent saccharides.

Cyclotetraglucose is naturally found in sake lees. It is sediment that forms during the production of rice wine, in sake itself, and in the cells of Saccharomyces cerevisiae. For the first time, cyclotetraglucose has been synthesized by treating alternant, which is a linear oligosaccharide, with alternanase.

In a large scale production, it is mainly produced by the combined action of 6-GT and IMT; both of them are isolated from Sporosarcina globispora, on liquefied starch.

6.6.5. Isoamylase from Pseudomonas Amyloderamosa

The P. amyloderamosa isoamylase is a kind of extracellular enzyme that is mainly secreted by the production strain to the broth of fermentation. Then, the fermentation broth is purified and concentrated to acquire the isoamylase activity within a required range.

After that, isoamylase is formulated with maltose and glucose, and either glycerol octylate or sodium benzoate and glycerol n-caproate. The water is further added to regulate the activity of isoamylase. The preparation of isoamylase enzyme includes lower levels of lipase, cellulose, and protease activity.

There are two isoamylase products, "Isoamylase M" and "Isoamylase S." Both formulations have around 37% of added sugars, glucose, and maltose. Isoamylase M comprises 0.05% of each, glycerol n-caproate and glycerol octylate, whereas Isoamylase S contains sodium benzoate as a substitute for glycerol fatty acid esters.

The preparation of isoenzyme is proposed for the use in the production of food ingredients from starch, comprising maltose, glucose syrup, trehalose, maltitol, cyclodextrins, and resistant starch. The preparation of isoamylase enzyme complies with the General Specifications and Considerations for Enzyme Preparations Used in Food Processing. Isoamylase from P. amyloderamosa was primarily recognized and described by Harada et al., (1968). Its physicochemical, as well as molecular characteristics, were then clarified and defined in numerous publications.

Isoamylase has an optimum pH at 3.0–4.0 and an optimum temperature at 52°C. The enzyme mainly comprises 750 residues of amino acid and has a molecular weight of around 80 kDa. The 3-D structure of isoamylase was revealed by the X-ray structure analysis.

The activity of isoamylase is determined by protecting the enzyme with soluble waxy corn starch as a substrate in the presence of iodine for almost 30 minutes under standard conditions (pH = 3.5; 40°C) and calculating the reaction mixture absorbance at 610 nm.

Any change in the absorbance shows the level of hydrolysis of the substrate. The activity of isoamylase is measured in isoamylase activity units (IAU) per gram of the enzyme preparation. One IAU is defined as the quantity of isoamylase that upsurges absorbance of the reaction mixture by 0.008 in 30 minutes under standard conditions (pH = 3.5; 40°C).

6.6.6. Phospholipase A1 from Fusarium venenatum Expressed in Aspergillus oryzae

It is produced by the submerged fed-batch and pure culture fermentation of a GM strain of Aspergillus oryzae comprising the phospholipase A1 gene which is usually derived from Fusarium venenatum.

The enzyme is isolated from the broth of fermentation by the technique of filtration to eliminate the biomass and is concentrated by the technique of ultrafiltration or evaporation. The residual production microbes are eliminated from the enzyme concentrate by the process of germ filtration.

The eventual product is then formulated by using food-grade stabilizing as well as preserving agents. The activity of Phospholipase A1 is measured compared with a phospholipase standard by applying lecithin as a substrate.

Phospholipase A1 catalyzes the lecithin hydrolysis to Lyso-lecithin and free fatty acid. The evolved fatty acid is then titrated with 0.1 N sodium hydroxide under standard conditions of 8.0 pH. The activity of phospholipase A1 is usually determined as the rate of sodium hydroxide consumption during the neutralization of the fatty acid. It is expressed in Lecitase units (LEU) relative to a Lecitase (phospholipase) standard.

6.6.7. Sodium Iron (III) Ethylenediaminetetraacetate

The synonyms of Sodium Iron (III) Ethylenediaminetetraacetate are Ferric sodium edetate, sodium iron EDTA, sodium feredetate. Its chemical names comprise Sodium [[N, N'-ethanediylbis [N-(carboxymethyl) glycinato]] (4-)] ferrate (1-); sodium [(ethylenedinitrilo) tetraacetato] ferrate (1-); Sodium iron (III) ethylenediaminetetraacetate. It is a powder of light yellow colour, which is stable and not even affected by the storage.

Usually, Ethylenediaminetetraacetic acid, iron (III) sodium salt hydrate (Sodium iron EDTA hydrate, EDTA ferric sodium salt hydrate) is instantly available in most volumes. High purity, submicron, and nanopowder forms may be taken into account.

The American Elements produces various standard grades when relevant, comprising Mil-Spec (military grade); Food, Agricultural, and Pharmaceutical Grade; ACS, Reagent, and Technical Grade; Optical Grade, USP and EP/BP (European Pharmacopoeia/British Pharmacopoeia) and trails appropriate testing standards of ASTM. Custom and typical packaging are also available. Extra technical research and safety information is present as is a Reference Calculator for changing the applicable units of measurement.

6.6.8. Branching Glycosyltransferase from Rhodothermus obamensis Expressed in Bacillus subtilis

Branching glycosyltransferase is made by the process of pure culture fermentation of a GM strain of Bacillus subtilis comprising a synthetic gene coding for branching glycosyltransferase from Rhodothermus obamensis.

Bacillus subtilis is a Gram-positive bacterium that is extensively distributed in nature and is measured to be non-toxigenic as well as non-pathogenic. It has a long history of use in enzyme production which is further used in food processing, together with enzymes from genetically engineered strains.

It has been granted a Qualified Presumption of Safety status by the European Food Safety Authority (EFSA) in the year 2008. Originally, the gene encoding branching glycosyltransferase was cloned from Rhodothermus obamensis, which is a thermophilic bacterium isolated from a marine hydrothermal vent.

Depending upon the sequence of amino acids in branching glycosyltransferase that is translated from the Rhodothermus obamensis gene, a synthetic gene was framed that converts branching glycosyltransferase with the same sequence of amino acid as that of the native Rhodothermus obamensis enzyme.

Subsequently, the gene was placed under deoxyribonucleic acid (DNA) regulatory sequences obtained from numerous Bacillus species and inserted into the Bacillus subtilis host strain JA1343 by the process of transformation. The chloramphenicol resistance gene (cat) was utilized in the transformation as a selectable marker, but it was then elucidated to make the production strain marker-free.

6.7. QUALITATIVE METHOD OF EVALUATION

6.7.1. Thin-Layer Chromatography

Thin-layer chromatography is a method for examining the mixtures by separating the components present in the mixture. It can be applied to determine the number of components in a given mixture, the identity of the component, and the purity of the component. By perceiving the look of a specific product or the loss of a reactant, it can also be utilized to monitor the growth of a reaction.

It is a kind of sensitive technique as it can analyze even microgram (0.000001 g) quantities and takes very less amount of time for analysis (i.e., around 5–10 minutes). It mainly consists of three key steps – spotting, development, and visualization (Figure 6.4).

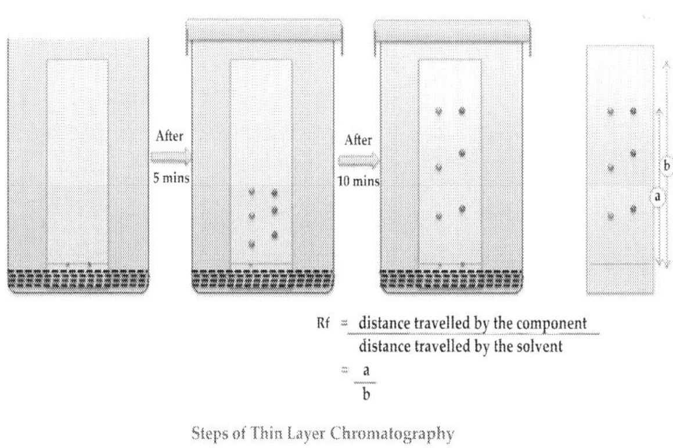

Figure 6.4. Thin layer chromatography.

Source: https://microbenotes.com/thin-layer-chromatography/

First of all, the sample which needs to be analyzed is dissolved in a volatile solvent to produce a dilute solution. In the process of spotting, a micro pipette is used to transfer a very small amount of the dilute solution to one end of a TLC plate.

The solvent of spotting quickly evaporates, leaving behind a spot of the material. The process of development mainly comprises placing the bottom of a TLC plate into a narrow pool of a development solvent, which then moves up to the plate by capillary action.

As the solvent moves up to the plate, it travels over the original spot. A major competition is organized between the silica gel plate and the development solvent for the spotted material. The polar silica gel attempts to hold the spot in its novel place and the solvent attempts to transfer the spot along with it as it moves up the plate.

The consequence majorly depends upon the balance amongst three polarities- that of the development solvent, TLC plate, and the spot material. If the development solvent is polar, the spot will move from its original location.

Distinct components present in the original spot, consisting of different polarities, will move diverse distances from the location of the original spot and make a separate spot. When the solvent has almost moved to the top of the TLC plate, the plate is then removed, and the solvent is marked with a pencil. Subsequently, the solvent is permitted to evaporate.

Visualization of the coloured components is very simple. The spots can be observed directly after the development. As most of the components are colourless, a method of visualization is extremely required. The silica gel present on the TLC plate is filled with a fluorescent material that eventually glows under ultraviolet (UV) light. A spot will then hinder the fluorescence and look like a dark spot on a glowing background.

Under the UV light, the spots can be sketched with a pencil to mark the locations. The second method of visualization is done by placing the TLC plate into the vapors of iodine for just a few minutes. In this case, organic components will form a dark-coloured complex with iodine.

It is considered to be a good practice of using at least two techniques of visualization. The retention factor (Rf) value is used to enumerate the movement of components along with the TLC plate. Rf value is defined as the equal distance moved by the component divided by the distance moved by the solvent. The Rf value is between zero and one, always.

An analysis of TLC might be briefed as, "Using a silica gel plate as well as ethyl acetate as the development solvent, unknown mixture X exhibited three spots having Rf value of 0.12, 0.25, and 0.87."

Comparing these Rf values with the Rf values of the known compound might allow an uncertain recognition to be made. If a development solvent of high polarity is used, all of the components present in the mixture will move along the solvent, and there will be no separation. The Rf value will be very large.

If the solvent used has a low polarity, the components will not move as required, and the separation will not take place. This time, the Rf value will be very small. Practically, mixtures of solvent or different solvents are tried till a good separation is detected. Normally, an effective solvent provides Rf's in the range of 0.3–0.7.

6.8. QUANTITATIVE METHOD OF EVALUATION

6.8.1. High-Pressure Liquid Chromatography

High-pressure liquid chromatography or High-performance liquid chromatography (HPLC) is a specific kind of column chromatography. This is generally used in the field of biochemistry to separate, recognize, and enumerate the active compounds.

It mainly employs a column that grasps the packing material, and it is known as the stationary phase, a pump that moves the mobile phase by the column, and a detector that depicts the retention time of the molecules. The retention time majorly varies based on the interactions or links between the stationary phase, the used solvent, and the molecules being identified.

The sample which is required to be analyzed is inserted into the stream of the mobile phase into a very small volume. This is retarded by explicit physical or chemical interactions with the stationary phase. The amount of retardation usually depends on the nature of the analyte present as well as the composition of the mobile and stationary phases.

The time at which an analyte comes out of the column is known as the retention time. The solvents that are commonly used in this process are any miscible combinations of water or organic liquids. The most common are acetonitrile and methanol.

Separation has been done to differentiate the composition of the mobile phase at the time of analysis, and this is called a gradient elution. The gradient splits the mixture of analytes as a function of the affinity of the analyte for the present mobile phase. The selection of solvents, gradients, and additives depending on the nature of the analyte as well as the stationary phase (Figure 6.5).

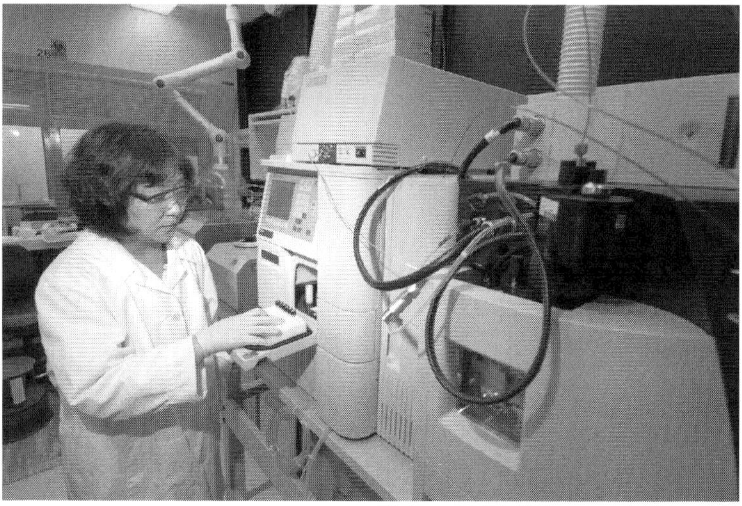

Figure 6.5. A research biologist Hui-Ping Chen, preparing a high-performance liquid chromatography.

Source: http://www.publicdomainfiles.com/show_file.php?id=13518558625346

6.8.1.1. Types of HPLC

- *Normal Phase Chromatography*: It is also known as NP-HPLC. This technique separates the analytes depending upon their polarities. NP-HPLC utilizes a polar stationary phase as well as a non-polar stationary phase. The polar analyte interacts with the polar stationary phase and gets retained by it. The strength of adsorption increases with increasing the polarity of an analyte, and the interaction between the polar stationary phase and polar analyte increases the time of elution.
- *Reversed-Phase Chromatography (RPC):* Reversed-phase high-pressure liquid chromatography (RP-HPLC or RPC) includes a non-polar stationary phase and an aqueous, discreetly polar mobile phase. RP-HPLC works on the principle of hydrophobic

interactions. The hydrophobic interactions result from the repulsive forces between a polar eluent, the non-polar stationary phase, and the relatively non-polar analyte.

The binding of the stationary phase and the analyte is directly proportional to the contact surface area near the segment of the analyte molecule upon bonding with the ligand present in the aqueous eluent.

- *Size Exclusion Chromatography*: Also known as gel filtration chromatography or gel permeation chromatography. It separates the particles depending upon the size of the particles. It is very significant for determining the tertiary as well as quaternary structure of proteins and amino acids. This method is extensively used for the determination of the molecular weight of polysaccharides.
- *Ion Exchange Chromatography*: In this, the retention is based on the interaction between charged sites and solute ions bound to the stationary phase. Ions of a similar charge are omitted out. This kind of chromatography is majorly used in the exchange of ligand, purification of water, chromatography of proteins, high-pH anion-exchange chromatography of oligosaccharides and carbohydrates, etc.
- *Bio-Affinity Chromatography*: In bio-affinity chromatography, the separation is based upon the specific reversible interaction of ligands and proteins. Ligands are covalently linked to the solid support on a matrix, holds the protein with interaction to the column-bound ligands.

Proteins that are bound to a bio-affinity column can be eluted in two ways:

- Bio-specific elution: Enclosure of free ligand in the elution buffer which contends with column bound ligand; and
- A specific elution: Change in salt, pH, etc. which fades the interaction of the protein with a column-bound substrate.

Due to the specificity of the interaction, bio-affinity chromatography can affect in a high purification in only a single step.

6.8.1.2. Instrumentation

- *Injection of the Sample*: Samples are injected by using different kinds of injectors. The sample can only be injected when the mobile phase is stopped, or it is flowing. An advanced rotary valve along with a loop injector can be used to produce desirable results.

- *The Detector:* There are numerous ways of detecting the substance when it passes through the column. UV spectroscopy detects the specific components of a substance. Various organic compounds absorb UV light of distinct wavelengths. The amount of light that is absorbed will depend upon the amount of a specific compound that is moving through the beam during that time.
- *Interpreting the Output from the Detector*: The output is usually recorded as a series of peaks. The peaks represent the compound that is moving through the detector and absorbing the UV light. The area present under the peaks is directly proportional to the amount of the compound to be identified, which is passed through the device detector. This area can be automatically calculated by the computer, which is linked to the display.

6.9. IDENTIFICATION AND ESTIMATION OF SYNTHETIC FOOD COLOURS

6.9.1. Chromatographic Separation of the Unknown Colour Mixture

The reagents that are needed for the separation of the colour mixture are 1% sodium chloride solution, NaCl 0.1% solutions of FD & C certified colours.

The process usually requires chromatography paper (Whatman No. 1 or equivalent), 600 mL beaker, 10 cm x 20 cm Capillary tubes, plastic wrap (Saran Wrap or similar) or watch glass to cover the beaker. The food colour standard solutions comprise 0.1% solutions of current, permitted, FD & C colours. The method starts with taking a sheet of chromatographic paper. Draw a line with a pencil of about 1 cm from the bottom of the sheet. With the help of a capillary tube, capillary-tipped dropper, or pointed glass rod, apply a small drop of the unknown colour mixture on the line drawn with a pencil, near the center of the chromatographic paper.

Mark the paper at the top, just above the spot with an X to indicate the unknown colour mixture. If the spot appears to be very small or very light in colour, make it darker by dropping another spot of colour directly on top of the dry first spot.

If the spot still appears to be very light in colour, extra spots can be made on the top of the previous dried spot. Spot the paper with every FD & C colour allowing around 2.0 cm least distance between each different spot.

Note the identity of every colour at the top of the paper above every spot. Add 1% NaCl solution in a 600 ml beaker. Bend the spotted paper in a cylindrical shape, put the ends together, and staple them. Place the chromatographic paper into the beaker and make sure that the spots are not below the level of solvent, and the paper is not touching the sides of the beaker (Figure 6.6).

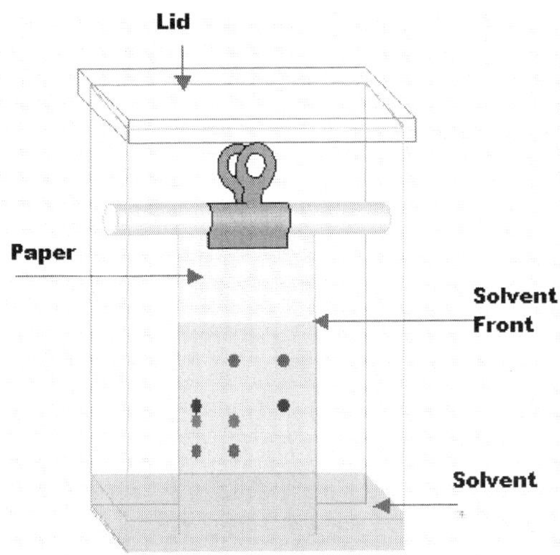

Figure 6.6. Paper chromatography.

Source: https://owlcation.com/stem/What-is-Paper-Chromatography-and-How-does-it-Work

Cover the beaker by using plastic wrap. Allow the solvent to move up the paper. This will require 15 to 35 minutes. Then, remove the paper from the beaker, open it, and mark the solvent front using a pencil. Put the chromatography paper on a paper towel to dry.

Measure and record the average distance from the origin to the solvent front as well as the distance each spot moved from the origin. Conclude the Rf values for each spot in the unknown mixture and for each of the FD & C colours that were used.

The Rf values for the components present in an unknown mixture will be equivalent for the same component in the FD & C known colours. By matching the colour as well as the Rf value of each of the spots, the identity of the colours extracted from the food can be easily determined.

REFERENCES

1. Benford, D., (2019). Carrageenan and Processed Eucheuma Seaweed (Addendum) (JECFA Food Additives Series 48). Retrieved from: http://www.inchem.org/documents/jecfa/jecmono/v48je08.htm (Accessed on 14 May 2019).
2. Ethylenediaminetetraacetic acid, iron (III) sodium salt hydrate | American Elements ®. Retrieved from: https://www.americanelements.com/ethylenediaminetetraacetic-acid-iron-iii-sodium-salt-hydrate-149022-26-4 (Accessed on 14 May 2019).
3. Food and Agricultural Organization, (1999). Sodium Iron (III) Ethylenediaminetetraacetate, Trihydrate [eBook] (p. 4). Retrieved from: http://www.fao.org/fileadmin/user_upload/jecfa_additives/docs/Monograph1/Additive-411.pdf (Accessed on 14 May 2019).
4. Food and Drug Administration, (2019). Human Studies [eBook] (p. 9). Retrieved from: https://www.fda.gov/downloads/Food/GuidanceRegulation/UCM078753.pdf (Accessed on 14 May 2019).
5. Katz, D., (1997). The Extraction and Identification of Artificial Food Colours [eBook] (p. 7). Retrieved from: http://www.chymist.com/Chromatography%20food%20colours.pdf (Accessed on 14 May 2019).
6. Kawamura, Y. Cyclotetraglucose and Cyclotetraglucose Syrup [eBook] (p. 10). Food and Agricultural Organization. Retrieved from: http://www.fao.org/fileadmin/templates/agns/pdf/jecfa/cta/68/Cyclotetraglucose.pdf (Accessed on 14 May 2019).
7. Malviya, R., Bansal, V., Kumar, S. P., & Pal, O., (2010). High-Performance Liquid Chromatography: A Short Review. Retrieved from: https://www.researchgate.net/publication/235987484_High_performance_liquid_chromatography_A_short_review (Accessed on 14 May 2019).
8. Mepham, B., (2011). Food additives: An ethical evaluation. British Medical Bulletin, 99(1), 7–23. doi: 10.1093/bmb/ldr024.
9. Olempska-Beer, Z. Asparaginase from Aspergillus oryzae Encoded by the Asparaginase Gene from Aspergillus oryzae [eBook] (p. 7). Food and Agricultural Organization. Retrieved from: http://www.fao.org/fileadmin/templates/agns/pdf/jecfa/cta/68/Asparaginase_from_A_oryzae.pdf (Accessed on 14 May 2019).

10. Olempska-Beer, Z., (2006). Isoamylase from Pseudomonas Amyloderamosa [eBook] (p. 6). Food and Agricultural Organization. Retrieved from: http://www.fao.org/fileadmin/templates/agns/pdf/jecfa/cta/68/Isoamylase.pdf (Accessed on 14 May 2019).
11. Pressman, P., Clemens, R., Hayes, W., & Reddy, C., (2017). Food Additive Safety. Toxicology Research and Application, 1, 239784731772357. doi: 10.1177/2397847317723572.
12. Rao, M. Acidified Sodium Chlorite (ASC) [eBook] (p. 12). Food and Agricultural Organization. Retrieved from: http://www.fao.org/fileadmin/templates/agns/pdf/jecfa/cta/68/Acidified_Sodium_Chlorite.pdf (Accessed on 14 May 2019).
13. Spielmann, H., (2002). Animal use in the safety evaluation of chemicals: Harmonization and emerging needs. ILAR Journal, 43(1), S11–S17. doi: 10.1093/ilar.43.suppl_1.s11.
14. Thin Layer Chromatography. [eBook] (p. 7). Retrieved from: https://people.chem.umass.edu/samal/269/tlc.pdf (Accessed on 14 May 2019)

Chapter 7

Information Resources in Toxicology

CONTENTS

7.1. INTRODUCTION

Toxicology information systems have progressed very rapidly. It has been changed from initial library-based bibliographic tools to progressive packages that are using sophisticated computer and telecommunication technologies.

These Toxicology information systems have grown simultaneously with the fast development of the science of toxicology itself. Bibliographic files characterize the very first efforts to handle the toxicology literature with the help of online retrieval. These bibliographic files can be TOXLINE (Figure 7.1).

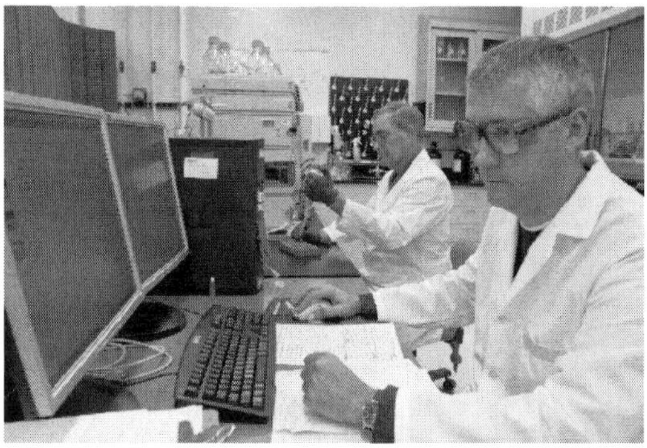

Figure 7.1. Toxicology has seen a rise in information resources with the help of technology.

Source: https://upload.wikimedia.org/wikipedia/commons/7/77/Toxicology_Research_at_FDA_%28NCTR_1387%29_%286008497229%29.jpg

The succeeding methods applied the use of computers to deliver the literature-derived data. This is similar to the case of HSDB or RTECS databanks, or to take the data directly from the laboratory. Many progressive systems are making use of the computational and analytical approaches to mine the knowledge from the laboratory data to forecast outcomes.

Many issues give rise to toxicity information. There exist social concerns about hazardous substances that are revealed in legislation and regulations. These social issues have been accountable for the generation of much toxicity information and the impetus to thoroughly collect and distribute these toxicity data.

The Scientific or technical progress in the subjects like molecular biology, chemistry, and bioinformatics are in combination with advances in information technologies. These scientific progress is also influencing the supply of toxicology information.

It has been observed that the amount of information has increased intensely since the last years. With the increase in information, it has become more accessible and current as compared to the past few years. The field must increase to the challenge of encouragement of data accessibility, endorsing data standards, and guaranteeing the quality of the data. This is done to derive meaning from the heap of data and information.

From the past three-decade years, the field of toxicology has observed extraordinary growth. This explosion in subject matter has arisen mainly from social issues and is coordinated by equally rapid technological invention as well as scientific advancement. This has brought about a serendipitous marriage between toxicology information and advanced systems. This further organizes, analyzes, and distributes this information.

As an applied science, toxicology tries to find the protect biological system that is against the unwanted effects from contact to agents that are damaging. Before the era of the 1960s, toxicology was considered a sub-discipline of pharmacology. At that time, toxicology paid its consideration to the protection of the prevailing and proposed pharmaceutical and consumer products.

Many factors have forested toxicology closer to the environmental problems. Though there exist environmental disasters all over the year 1950s and the year 1960 that have edged toxicology closer to the front of environmental problems. The environmental disasters were like the mercury poisonings in Minamata and 'killer fog' in London.

There was a conference that was held in the year 1960, which was titled 'Problems in Toxicology.' This conference has brought the different scientists all together to address not only food, drug, and cosmetic control but this conference also paid attention to address the environmental chemicals, pesticides, industrial chemicals, radioactive materials, and many more. The main objective of this conference was that 'toxicity is suddenly upon us as a social problem.'

It took more than two years for the publication of Silent Spring in the year 1962. This publication made the public aware of the dangers that are linked with the uncontrolled production and the usage of thousands of chemicals. Toxicology became caught up in the tide of the environmental movement.

Toxicology came out from under pharmacology's shadow, and it started to grow into a full-scale discipline of its own. One of the main features of toxicology is its multidisciplinary nature. This multidisciplinary nature is to draw upon the progress in chemistry, biology, genetics, statistics, and other sciences.

In addition to this, toxicology has also laid several numbers of subspecialties of its own. Some of these subspecialties are ecotoxicology (ECOTOX), forensic toxicology, veterinary toxicology, clinical toxicology. The demand for along with the supply of toxicology information has grown simultaneously as the discipline has grown.

There are several numbers of varied groups that have the requirement for toxicology information. They acquire toxicology information from research scientists and pharmaceutical drug developers to occupational hygienists and members of the public. The toxicology information that is used by the different users is varied as the type of users.

This toxicology information is used to improve understanding of how environmental agents have an impact on the biological, chemical, and genetic mechanisms to evaluate the risk of chemical exposure to handle the regulatory decision-making. This is done to ensure effective and safe drug development, which then diminish or eliminate public and occupational exposures to hazardous substances. Every application drives the type of information that is required. So, the toxicological information is converted into too many forms. The raw laboratory data that are quantitative, qualitative, and descriptive links to chemical properties, physical properties, toxic endpoints, etc. The field data capture incidence statistics, exposure data, hazard monitoring, accidental release levels, etc. On the other hand, there are visual images that are in the form of pathology slides, gene expression data, histochemical profiles, etc. The Textual content from statutes/regulatory details, articles, technical reports, etc. The demand for and supply of toxicology information has been driven by the interplay among three influential forces. These three influential forces are regulatory measures, scientific progress, and technological advances.

7.2. TECHNOLOGICAL INNOVATION IN THE INFORMATION RESOURCES IN TOXICOLOGY

The leaps that were observed in computing speed, hard disk size, and memory space were first of their kind in the history of information resources of the food toxicology have helped in the storage, retrieval, analysis, and distribution of ever-growing volumes of data and information.

This resulted in the transformation of the paper-based tools of card catalogues and indexes into fully searchable databases. Telecommunications and digital networks form the backbone of the Internet and the World Wide Web. They are considered as the pillar of the internet. They make it likely to share a wealth of information not only locally, but also it can share the information globally without any restrictions.

Web browsers, search engines, subject directories, and hypertext support information retrieval on the World Wide Web. Many features have helped in social networking. Electronic mail, listservs, instant messaging, and discussion groups enable social networking and person-to-person communication.

On the other hand, the Wireless communication networks are allowing portable, handheld devices to be used in the applications. These handheld devices can be used in a diversity of applications. The National Library of Medicine (NLM) has gone over a few of this toxicology-related PDA software (Figure 7.2).

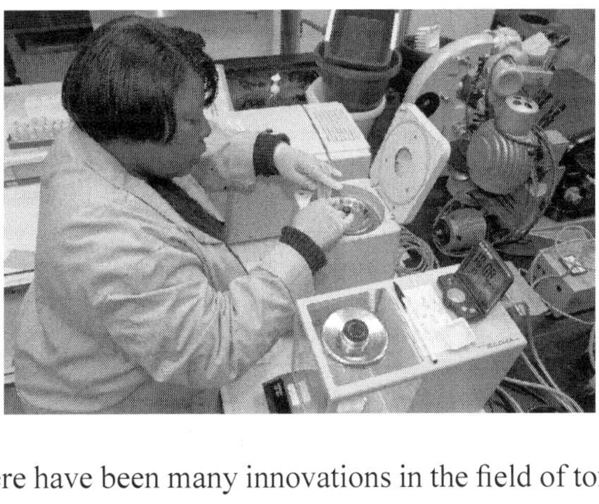

Figure 7.2. There have been many innovations in the field of toxicology in past few years.

Source: https://farm7.staticflickr.com/6150/6008495935_4aa31ab653_b.jpg

In addition to this, the analytical tools and instruments have more and more become integrated with computing systems. These tools are combined with the computer systems to create a seamless flow of capturing, and also, helps in the storage of information for the examination and interpretation of the data.

There was one earlier system that was developed around the year 1980. This was established by the National Center for Toxicological Research. This system allowed the collection, processing, and analysis of large-scale, rodent-based tests.

On a much larger scale, Xybion's PATH/TOX system joins in toxicology, pharmaceutical, histology, pathology, necropsy, and other laboratory activities into a united wide-ranging data acquisition and management system.

These kinds of data-collecting and -processing systems are generally planned for support of research and testing inside an organization. It is to be noted that the resultant data banks are not generally available to outsiders. This resultant data bank is not available to the people outside the organization.

Though, the beginning of the Internet and the growing expectations of many scientists or researchers are slowly encouraging the availability of open data. Some instances of databases that helped in making the research results publicly accessible include the various NCBI Entrez molecular biology databases such as GenBank and the Swiss Institute of Bioinformatics ExPASy server for proteomics.

These centralized databases provide a web interface for any researcher or scientist to upload data and perform queries. The other form of open access data sharing is with the help of federated data sites. In federated data sites, each facility maintains its site. On the other hand, the central interface permits the researchers to search across multiple resources.

The Biomedical Informatics Research Network (BIRN) was developed in this mode. This was originated by the National Institutes of Health. The BIRN that is BIRN is a virtual community that is geologically dispersed. This consists of shared resources that are providing great potential to improve the analysis and treatment of disease.

These advancements in technology have created a paradigm move in scientific discovery. The greatest influence of these advancements is noticeable in the generation, utilization, and dissemination of exponential volumes of information.

It has been observed that the ironic consequence is that advancement in technology has given a rise to an ever-expanding volume of data. Thus, there is a need for faster and more powerful information systems to be able to manage it all.

But more knowingly, technology has rooted itself into the core of the scientific research process. The processes that are influencing the approaches that are used, the rate of progress that is accomplished, and the track of research effort. The discipline of toxicology is not resistant to the impact of the technology. It has been observed the behaviour of toxicology has been reorganized with an improved dependence on technology-driven approaches.

7.3. HISTORY OF INFORMATION RESOURCES IN TOXICOLOGY

The main three factors have generated an overabundance of reports, articles, toxicity tests, etc. Afterward, it helps in promoting a requirement for information systems to collect, organize, manage, and examine the arrival of data and information which is coming from these sources.

7.3.1. What Is An Information System?

At the present times, people seem to believe that an information system requires computing technology the information system may be 'automated or manual and comprises people, machines, and/or methods to 'capture, transmit, store, retrieve, manipulate, or display information to serve a specific purpose.'

The proposed purpose of the information system describes the category of data, structure, and interface to be used in the system. At the time of dealing with the hybrid nature of toxicology, an added challenge occurs of handling the information from diverse disciplines, each of this with its terminology, datasets, methodologies, and technologies.

7.3.2. Early Toxicology Information Systems

The history of literature of Toxicology dates back as early as 1500 BC with the Ebers Papyrus. It is defined as the effects of poisons. Since the year 1930, the discipline did not find its publication voice with the Sammlung von Vergiftungsfällen.

An editorial published in the year 1959 stated that the journal was needed because 'toxicology is emerging as a scientific discipline and that there is a requirement for centralization of toxicology data. This editorial was stated in the first issue of the English journal Toxicology and Applied Pharmacology.

Till the year the 1970s, the printed matter and professional meetings were the main sources for the distribution of information in the field. The subsequent growth in publishing has given rise to the increased demand for toxicology information because of the regulations and researcher interest. On the other hand, this encouraged the need for a means to manage and keep the record of the literature. Therefore, indexing and abstracting tools were developed. These tools were developed to capture the wealth of information that is summarized in the journal articles. There are many dependable standards such as Biological Abstracts, Chemical Abstracts, Excerpta Medica, and Index Medicus that offer a way of tracking toxicology literature of toxicology. Although these dependable standards provide a limited way as compared to modern standards.

It has been observed that there were no information systems that were devoted to serve the toxicologist, to pull all together and make readily available the wide-ranging data. This wide-ranging data was being generated by increased testing and appearing in an increasing array of publications (Figure 7.3).

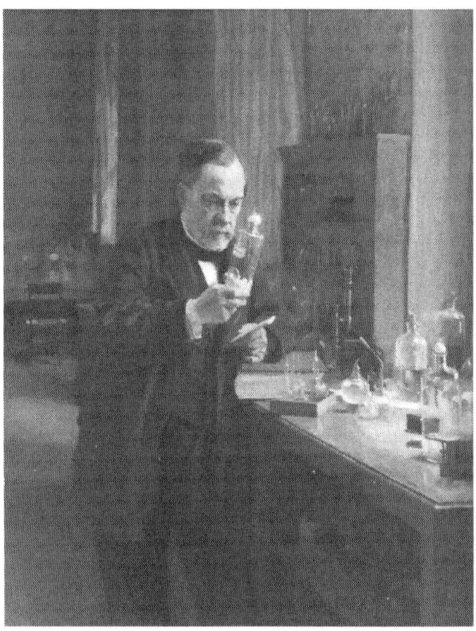

Figure 7.3. The information resources in toxicology dates back to many centuries.

Source: https://upload.wikimedia.org/wikipedia/commons/3/3c/Albert_Edelfelt_-_Louis_Pasteur_-_1885.jpg

One of the main documents that are providing a vision into the broadcasting of toxicology information was the 1966 Report of the United States President's Science Advisory Committee. This United States President's Science Advisory Committee is entitled 'Handling of Toxicological Information,' known here as the PSAC Report. The PSAC Panel stated its concern regarding the dispersion of toxicological information over a huge area of the published journal literature, published, and unpublished reports, and unpublished information files of industrial companies and government agencies.

The main finding of the panel was that 'there exists an urgent requirement for a much more synchronized and more complete computer-based file of toxicological information as compared to any other that is available at present available. And, after that the access to this file be more usually available to all those legitimately those who require such information' The recommendations of the PSAC Paneled, in the year 1967, to the formation of the Toxicology Information Program (TIP) at the NLM.

7.4. CURRENT TOXICOLOGICAL PRACTICES

In the sight of the pace of advances in the biological sciences, it may happen as a wonder to those new in the field. It may happen as a miracle, especially for the students who are new graduates with an orientation toward molecular genetics. Molecular genetics is the principal of safety evaluation. This is defined by many scientists more than 50 years past still describe comparatively accurately current regulatory toxicological practice as it applies to the estimation of general organ and tissue damage (Figure 7.4).

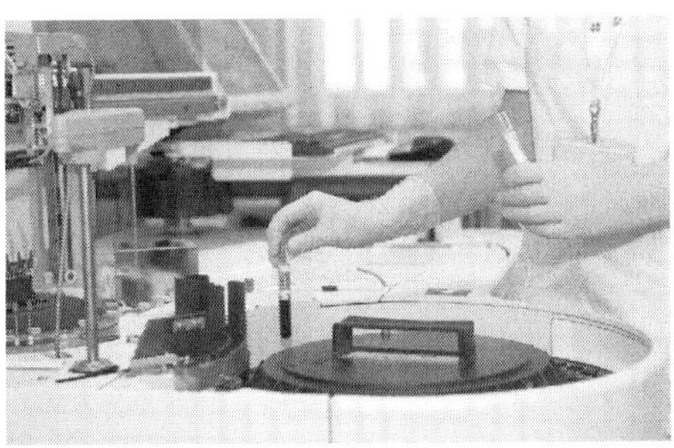

Figure 7.4. The current toxicological practices are based on complex use of the technology.

Source:https://cdn.pixabay.com/photo/2014/12/10/20/48/medic-563423_960_720.jpg

This historical method was extended upon in the classical review of Barnes and Denz. These historical tactics comprise of assessment of the impact of a substance on growth and tissue mass that is body and organ weights, this also includes measurements of serum biomarkers [aspartate aminotransferase (AST), alanine aminotransferase (ALT), alkaline phosphatase (ALP), etc.], hematological evaluation, examination of behaviour and appearance, as well as the histopathology assessment.

This historical method is fundamentally the approach. At the present time, this approach is practiced by the most important product industries. The industries that comprise the pharmaceutical and food industries.

Even though the toxicological practice has been constant as compared to the practices in the past few decades. This toxicology does not include the introduction of specialized tests for genetic and reproductive damage and some other special functional assessments. These special functional assessments are like the immunological, neurological, electrophysiological, and all indications are that the field is now poised for major change.

A glimpse at the program of current annual meetings of the Society of Toxicology, or the ever-increasing schedule of toxico- or pharmacogenomics meetings, leave behind the little uncertainty. This uncertainty is that toxicologists in industry, academia, and government are intensively estimating modern molecular technologies. As the people anticipate how these technologies may influence the practice that exists at the present times, the first thing to do is that the major elements of the current strategy should be considered. In essence, the in-vivo toxicological assessment of organ and tissue damage, comprises the assessment of three basic types of "biomarkers." These biomarkers specify adverse biological effects on the organism. There are three different types of markers that are used. These types of markers are:

- Function and homeostasis;
- Cell and tissue integrity; and
- Cell and tissue damage or damage-response.

The most important elements of this strategy are sound. But on the other hand, the biotechnology revolution has presented major opportunities to enhance the biomarkers that involve these three classes. The main focus is on the potential for improved biomarkers inside these three classes. These include both the molecular markers themselves, and it also includes the methodologies for monitoring those markers.

7.4.1. Opportunities for Improved Approaches to Toxicological Assessment

Some of the changes that are existing for improved toxicological assessment are created by the advances in molecular technologies and the enhanced knowledge of the molecular basis of tissue damage and response. This also comprises of the opportunities. These opportunities are for enhanced biomarkers, better technologies for monitoring biomarkers, and new laboratory models. These models also include human biochemical characteristics.

The instances of implementation of each of these opportunities already exist. Some many articles and papers pay attention to the influence of the recent revolution in genetics and biotechnology on strategies for the enhanced biomarker development and application, and also, on the assessment of the role of genetic variation in determining or modifying toxicological outcomes.

The new technologies of molecular biology are practically being used in several numbers of methods. They are applied in numerous ways to assess the function and structure of the major organ and tissue systems.

At present, most of the attention is focused on the ability of DNA microarrays to recognize either the inducible damage responses or shifts in gene expression patterns that are a trait of specific molecular insults to the cell.

This main focus is determined by the merging of two factors. These two factors comprise the accessibility of technology to take care of the expression of many genes at the same time using very small samples of DNA or RNA. On the other hand, the other factor is the newly developed knowledge that molecular evolution has given rise to specific inducible defence systems and regulatory control ways for significant cell functions.

There also includes other additional opportunities. These additional opportunities comprise the potential. The ability:

- To develop wide-ranging panel of biomarkers of cell and tissue integrity with the help of proteomic technologies.
- For one-to-one care of the functional pathways for the significant cell functions with the help of metabonomic technologies.
- For the development of mechanism-based models of human disease. This comprises the short-term models of carcinogenesis.
- To recognize genetic alterations that have given rise to human disease.

- For the use of imaging technologies to noninvasive monitoring.

7.5. APPLICATION OF INFORMATION RESOURCES IN TOXICOLOGY

In addition to the drawing from other disciplines, the toxicology information and its systems contribute to other fields also. There are many areas of application of information systems of toxicology. Some of them are used in environmental science, clinical medicine, drug development, occupational health, and public health.

7.5.1. Environmental Toxicology

The field of environmental toxicology provides insights into the passage of agents through the environment, and also this field of toxicology tells about how those agents may harm flora, fauna, and the broader ecosystem.

There exists some information that is very critical for the ECOTOX systems. This information comprises of the chemical as well as species-specific. The chemical property databases of significance comprise CHEMFATE and BIODEG. Both of these abstract empirical data on a chemical's environmental fate and biodegradation from the bibliographic literature (Figure 7.5).

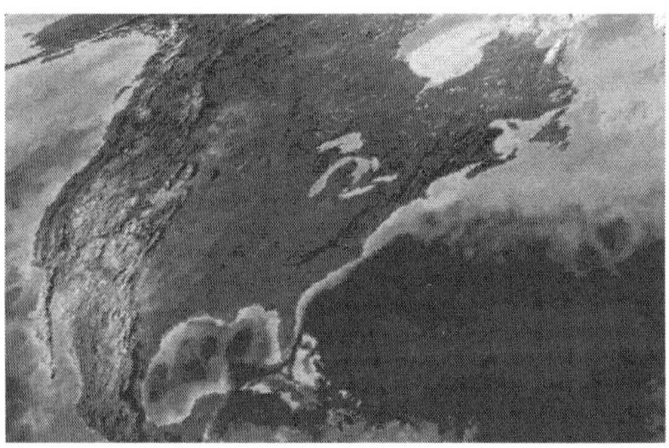

Figure 7.5. The most important field of application of toxicology is the environmental toxicology.

Source: https://upload.wikimedia.org/wikipedia/commons/2/2d/NorthAmericaCycle_Small.gif

It has been observed that the ecotoxicity databases are more often used for risk assessment, chemical screening and ranking, and predictive modeling. In the year 1995, the EPA's ECOTOX database was established as a single portal for the process of searching and recovering toxicity data from the AQUIRE that is the aquatic life, PHYTOTOX that is terrestrial plants, and also from TERRETOX that is wildlife databases.

In the beginning, this data was easily made available to the users of the government. This was done through the help of telnet. On the other hand, it became available openly when a web-based interface was launched in the year 2000.

At this time, ECOTOX comprises more than 320,000 individual effect records abstracted from 17,195 peer-reviewed publications. This publication or newspaper is representing over 7,800 chemicals and 5,300 aquatic and terrestrial species.

ECOTOX also enables the distribution of the data through the option of ASCII that is the American National Standard Code for Information Interchange delimited file formats. The Environmental Residue-Effects Database (ERED) is a joint EPA–US Army Corp of Engineers effort that is abstracted from the literature. This literature stated the connections between tissue contaminant concentrations and toxic responses. For instance, behavioural, biochemical, cellular, reproductive, etc.

The database put a cover on the literature that was published from the year 1964 to the year 2001. It also includes more than 3,463 records that are abstracted from near about 700 publications or newspapers. This is covering more than 222 compounds and 188 aquatic species.

There exist two expert systems, IPEST, and POCER (Pesticide Occupational and Environmental Health Risk Indicator). These systems estimate the ecological influence of a pesticide for a specific field crop on groundwater, surface water, air, soil, and humans.

Geographic information systems (GIS) have found new uses in the field of risk assessment and exposure. The U.S. Environmental Protection Agency has established a GIS-based application. This application joins together the wind speed, pesticide application rates, and other parameters to evaluate the possibility of non-target areas. The area that is being exposed to a chemical hazard, which plants species would be more sensitive, and monitoring the possible sites for carrying out the field surveys or monitoring.

7.5.2. Clinical Toxicology

In the terms of clinical practice, the application of toxicology information is typically is directed in the direction of treating patients who are going through the adverse effects from a toxic agent or pharmaceutical interaction.

In the early times, poison management information has been text-based. On the other hand, at the present times, the poison control centers and emergency physicians depend on online tools such as Micromedex POISINDEX. This system rapidly and accurately recognizes the ingredients that are present in thousands of commercial, biological, and pharmaceutical products. This system then provides information on clinical effects, the range of toxicity, and also it provides information on the treatment protocols.

Similar effects have been seen in the product named TOXBASE. TOXBASE a product of the UK National Poisons Information Service. This product is a longstanding poison and drug interaction database that has been used till the year 1998. Skyscape has established another tool. And this developed tool was made specifically for mobile use.

Its 5 Minute Toxicology Consult (5MTox) is a handheld form of the desktop download edition. It is geared toward the clinician who is in the need to quickly assess and treat a poisoned patient. There exists another system that is known as CliniTox. CliniTox is a computer-based decision support system that helps in providing veterinarians with the most current clinical toxicology information for poisoned farm animals. Users may search which is based on chemical, the kind of application, or clinical/pathological outcome.

7.5.3. Drug Discovery and Development

It had been observed that the combinatorial chemistry and high-throughput screening techniques have helped in catering to the phenomenal growth in the amount of potentially beneficial pharmacological compounds.

Until now, that increase in the number has not resulted in an increase in the new drug applications and effective acceptance by the FDA. The culprit of the high erosion rate is the loss of compounds to pass the toxicity testing.

The connection between predictive modeling, toxicogenomics, microscale computing, and chemoinformatics offers the opportunity to mine the important ADME Tox. Here ADME Tox refers to its absorption, distribution, metabolism, and excretion. This ADME Tox and pharmacokinetic data is mine to enhance a chemical's pharmacological properties and lessen its toxicity (Figure 7.6).

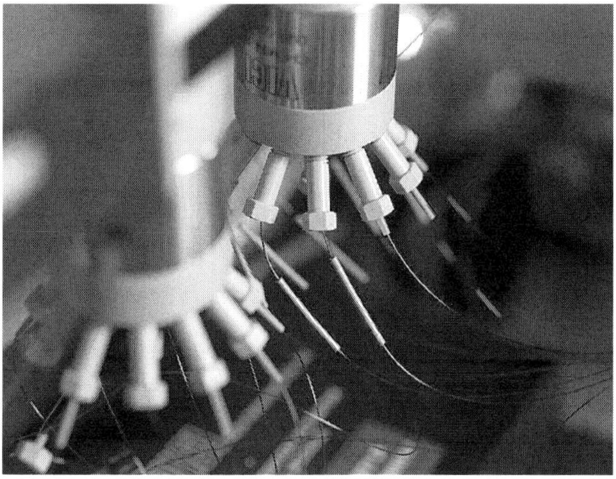

Figure 7.6. There are many important usages in the discovery of the drug.

Source: http://res.publicdomainfiles.com/pdf_view/197/14022892827853.jpg

Pharmacological data repositories include Wombat. Wombat is a database that comprises more than 136,000 chemical and 307,000 biochemical activity. The derivative of Wombat is Wombat PK, and which is also used for a similar purpose.

A clinical pharmacokinetic database comprises 643 drugs with human ADMETox outcomes. The application of microscale computing is the determination of the metabolic fate of a compound. This application of the determination of the metabolic fate of compounds is speeding up the drug discovery procedure by removing the toxic compounds at the initial or the preclinical phase of drug development.

The Metabolizing Enzyme Toxicology Assay Chip (MetaChip) can quickly and effectively measure a metabolic reaction of the drugs as if it was taking place in a human liver.

7.5.4. Occupational Health

To ensure the security of workers, there is the need of knowing the nature of chemical hazards and what to do in case of exposure. One of the initial beneficial resources was a reference book. This book is entitled Patty's Industrial Hygiene and Toxicology. At the present time, Patty's is available online as an e-book. This makes it much more available and easier to use for the users.

There exist two multi-file systems that integrate medical, chemical hazard, environmental, toxicological, regulatory, and risk information. The risk details comprise TOMES (Micromedex) and ExPub that are known as Expert Publishing. TOXNET's HAZMAP makes the connection of the jobs and hazardous tasks with occupational diseases and their systems.

At present times, the wireless information system makes use of mobile technology. The Wireless Information System for Emergency Responders that can also be written as WISER provides emergency personnel with the prepared information. For instance, the information can be substance identification, human health effects, containment advice, etc. This information helps the wireless information system to respond to hazardous material incidents.

There are several numbers of international efforts that are involved in providing chemical safety information. The International Program on Chemical Safety's INCHEM database provides up-to-date and peer-reviewed chemical safety publications or newspapers and database records.

The OECD's Environmental, Health, and Safety Program consist of a wide range of compiled databases. This database is related to high production volume chemicals, industrial chemical releases, among other issues.

7.5.5. Public Health

It has been observed that several numbers of information systems have been established. These information systems were specifically developed for public health professionals or the public directly. In January 2001, the Pew Environmental Health Commission issued the report 'America's Environmental Health Gap: Why the Country Needs a Nationwide Health Tracking Network' (Pew Environmental Health Commission, 2000).

The report specified that the current or present environmental health system is neither adequate nor it is well-organized, suggested the creation of a 'Nationwide Health Tracking Network for disease and exposures.

This resulted in the creation of the CDC's National Environmental Public Health Tracking Program. This program was created to track, monitor, and also it helped in associating the relationships among hazards, exposures, and health effects. Some websites served as a collection of their own as well as other government agencies' resources, databases, and programs. In the advancement of more public-oriented toxicology resources, the NLM's TEHIP has been a leader.

There exist four interesting databases that are very important for the public audience. These interesting databases comprise the Household Products Database (HPD), ToxTown, ToxMap, and Lact-Med. With the help of the HPD, the consumers can connect the consumer brand products with the known health effects that are related to their ingredients.

The information is abstracted from the product labels and Material Safety Data Sheets. ToxTown is an interactive website that helps in involving the public to gain knowledge about the interrelationship among chemicals, the environment, and public health.

It has been observed that the emphasis has been laid on the locations or sites wherein the people may be exposed to chemicals, and further information that is related to the nature and effects of the chemical is provided.

ToxMap is the website that makes use of geographic information system technology to generate local, state or national maps. In this, the Toxic emits the Inventory chemicals that have been released on-site into the air, water, or ground.

On the other hand, LactMed is of great importance for both clinicians and breastfeeding mothers about which drugs may be spread by breast milk. By the extraction from peer-reviewed literature, the data comprises several details. For instance, the information includes the maternal and infant levels of drugs, possible impact on breastfed infants and lactation, and alternate drugs to consider.

7.6. MODERN APPROACHES TO TOXICOLOGY

It has been observed that the public interest groups and grassroots organizations have also been contributing to the mass of toxicology information systems in the current years. Initially, the chemical Scorecard was launched by the Environmental Defence in the year 1998. The chemical scorecard provides local environmental information on the release of toxic chemicals from the neighbouring industrial facilities.

The site was transferred to Green Media Toolshed in the year 2005. The CHE Toxicant and Disease Database review the connection between the chemical contaminants and there exist near about 180 human diseases or conditions. Mainly the information is based on human epidemiological data. The Pesticide Action Network's also known as PANNA. It is an online

PAN Pesticides Database that sums up the human toxicity, ecotoxicity, and regulatory information from several numbers of sources on over 6,400 active ingredients in pesticides.

It is quite evident that the field of food toxicology is seeing an era of radical transformation. Many technological advances are capable of altering the methods that are being conventionally used in the information resources of food toxicology. The methods from which the data is generated and extracted, and the appearance of the food toxicology have allowed the conventional methods of study endpoints to face the levels of evolution. These levels of evolution have forced the conventional methods to gear up with the deeper levels of analytics and more deep insights into the information resources for food toxicology (Figure 7.7).

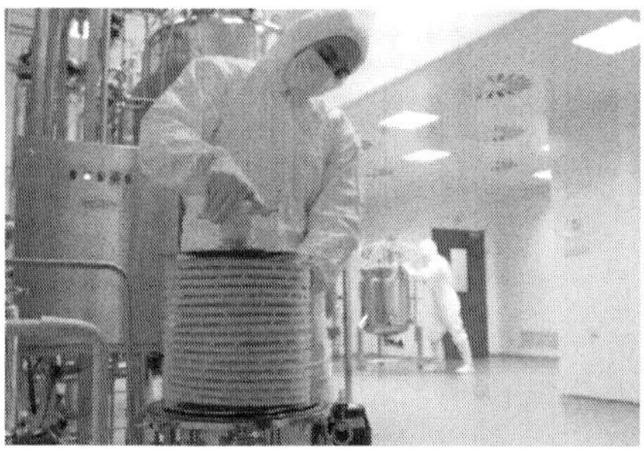

Figure 7.7. There are many advance methodologies that are being used in the toxicology.

Source: https://upload.wikimedia.org/wikipedia/en/1/11/Inside_Aryogen.jpg

The combination of modern experimental and computational ways offers the field of food toxicology a great capability for more effective, efficient, and dependable policies that can be used in the testing of food toxicology. However, with the advent of technology in the field of toxicology, a rise in the number of challenges and obstacles has been observed. The sudden and steep growth of the data, tools, and resources that are used in toxicology has a certain indication.

This means that it might be difficult to arrive at a decision on which of the chosen methodologies might perform the best. Similarly, the assessment of the reproducibility of the scientific discoveries requires the full authority to access the protocols and data that are being set for the systems of toxicology. Also, there is a need to build an effective system to manage the data that is extracted using the methodologies of toxicology.

Some many laboratories and institutes are working in the direction of the development of the range of new technologies, methodologies, and initiatives. This is being done in an attempt to progress in the field of toxicology. Apart from the progress, it is also important to address some of the challenges that are prevailing and are being faced by the community. Many articles are being used to describe some of the modern in vitro approaches to toxicology, as well as initiatives we are running to facilitate the verification of methods and conclusions and to enhance data sharing and scientific discovery.

7.6.1. Advances in In-Vitro Approaches to Toxicology

One of the most important events of toxicology in the twenty-first century is the development of more advanced in vitro models. These in vitro models are capable of offering new opportunities for physiologically relevant testing. Many models can diminish the necessity for animal testing.

Along with the reduction in animal testing, these models are capable of offering more cost-effective and results within a short time, as well as a better understanding of the biological processes that explain the fundamentals of toxicity.

The advances in the in-vitro approach to toxicology have many significant suggestions for the industry as well as for the regulatory bodies that are responsible for the scientific mistake of chemicals, pharmaceuticals, and many other consumer products.

At the present moment, some many observatories and laboratories have focused on developing a wide range of novel advanced in vitro techniques for the scientific assessment of reduced-risk products. The reduced-risk products are those products that contain non-combustible nicotine and tobacco products that can significantly diminish the individual risk and also reduce the population harm as compared to the harm that is inflicted by the cigarettes. Two unique methods allow the researchers to apply the information systems in toxicology techniques to get a better understanding and explore the information that is buried deep down in the layers of biological understanding. The two unique models are:

7.6.2. Three-Dimensional Organotypic Models

The three-dimensional organotypic models are used to evaluate the biological impact of the aerosol that is generated from reduced-risk products and the tobacco heating system. Some many studies and surveys have been

process as Industrial Methodology for Process Verification in Research, commonly known as the IMPROVER.

This method uses the principles of crowd-sourcing and cooperative opposition. The project is specifically designed as a set of open challenges on the scientific level. In this method, the methodologies and results are linked to particular scientific challenges. These scientific challenges are thoroughly scrutinized and reviewed without and biasing.

Industrial Methodology for Process Verification in Research, commonly known as the IMPROVER, is specifically created and designed to make sure that the reliability and reproducibility of the scientific results.

The main challenges in this method are:

- Many contributors are incorporated in the completion of the process, and all these contributors work at an individual level, thereby bringing independent methodologies and knowledge.
- Many different resolutions can be applied to various methods of a critically complex problem.
- Many different solutions can be applied in different combinations to identify the best-fit approach.
- Benchmarking is unbiased.
- The results and the conclusions are produced in the capability of being recreated and reproduced and thus can be used with a high degree of surety.

Till the present times, the method of Industrial Methodology of Process Verification in Research and the challenges that are being faced by this method have appeared at the verification and the identification of biomarkers of disease.

Along with the identification of the biomarker, this method explores the extent to which any biological processes are conserved across species, the inclusiveness of any biological network is being modeled, and the approximate value of the expression of the blood gene data.

7.6.5. Scientific Discovery and Data Sharing

In the field of toxicology, along with the different fields of biomedical sciences, the advancements in technology over the last few decades have led to an exponential growth in the process of data generation. Some observatories and laboratories are working in the interest of scientific discovery and to benefit and facilitate the capability of recreating the conclusions.

These laboratories believe the future of information resources in toxicology is held totally in the full disclosure of the data and reproducibility of this data. It is quite evident that, in present times, there are many complications and challenges for discovering and sharing large chunks of data. Majorly, the researchers working on the information resources in toxicology deal with large, multi-faceted, and extremely complex datasets.

So, it has become extremely important to create such a way that the data that has to be shared should be done by using such technologies and mechanisms that have a practical approach for the other scientists that are working in the same direction. The other scientists should be able to find and cross-check with the data that has been discovered and used earlier by their fellow scientists.

For the above-discussed reasons, some laboratories and observatories have launched a program INTERVALS. This program corresponds to the technology of an inhalation toxicology repository for the reduced-risk product data and research. The website which hosts this methodology provides the access to a complete and interpreted dataset. This kind of datasets that have been generated by the other scientists as a part of their development and evaluation of the datasets of the reduced-risk products.

This website has been designed to facilitate the recreation and reuse of the methodologies and data-sets practically. This helps in evaluating the reproducibility and the reliability of the scientific findings.

Along with access to the raw data, the facility of INTERVALS is also capable of providing the quality of metadata. This high-quality metadata can be utilized to describe the practical and experimentations. Apart from describing the experiments, this high-quality metadata can also be used for the processes of data production, data processing, and providing additional information that might prove relevant to the projects that are being proceeded simultaneously.

Many different technologies are being used for the extraction and the interpretation of these highly complex datasets. One of the most commonly used technologies, to extract and interpret the datasets with multiple levels of complexity, is the Garuda Technology. The Garuda technology helps in connecting a variety of the different databases of the INTERVALS, interlinking the various applications and the usage of the services that require a language-independent interface.

The usage of the INTERVALS allows the users to create and build flexible and customizable research and materials that help in creating a smooth workflow. Apart from the customizable interface, there are many modified tools by which it is very easy to visualize the data and then analyze the data required for the interpretation of the results of the work. The technology of the Garuda is an open platform that is controlled and driven by the community.

The Garuda technology is being used similarly and is aligned with the guidelines and the principles of transparency that are being used as the foundation of the INTERVALS platform. Eventually, the use of Garuda Technology that is being based on similar guidelines as that of the INTERVALS platform provides an opportunity to the researchers to use the data and perform the tasks of addition and extraction of the meaningful and useful information that is being stacked up on the large scale datasets with multilevel of complexity.

In particular, the platform of the INTERVALS was created and designed for usage in inhalation toxicology. But the concept of the INTERVALS platform can prove significant and can be used in many different areas. For example, these varied fields of applications are the calculation of pharmaceutical products, air-pollution risk management, and the current discoveries and innovations that are being done in the field of nanotechnology.

It is very essential that the usage of the INTERVALS platform can be seen in any field we're dealing with the huge set of data is required. Essentially, any field which deals with large and complex data could benefit from this approach as the issues concerning transparency, data reusability, and reproducibility is general across the sciences.

REFERENCES

1. Chemical Watch, (2018). Data and Toxicology: The Challenges Ahead. [online] Available at: https://chemicalwatch.com/70942/data-and-toxicology-the-challenges-ahead (Accessed on 14 May 2019).
2. Gosslau, A., (2016). Assessment of food toxicology. Food Science and Human Wellness, [online] 5(3), pp. 103–115. Available at: https://www.sciencedirect.com/science/article/pii/S2213453016300106.
3. Hoeng, J., & Peitsch, M., (2017). The Future of Toxicology: An Industry Case Study. [online] Drug discovery from technology networks. Available at: https://www.technologynetworks.com/drug-discovery/blog/the-future-of-toxicology-an-industry-case-study-294970 (Accessed on 14 May 2019).
4. MacGregor, J., (2003). The future of regulatory toxicology: Impact of the biotechnology revolution. Toxicological Sciences, [online] 75(2), pp. 236–248. Available at: https://doi.org/10.1093/toxsci/kfg197 (Accessed on 14 May 2019).
5. Pressman, P., Clemens, R., Hayes, W., & Reddy, C., (2017). Food additive safety. Toxicology Research and Application, [online] 1(2), p. 239784731772357. Available at: https://journals.sagepub.com/doi/full/10.1177/2397847317723572 (Accessed on 14 May 2019).
6. Schell, L., Gallo, M., & Cook, K., (2012). What's NOT to eat- Food adulteration in the context of human biology. US National Library of Medicine National Institutes of Health. [online] Available at: https://www.ncbi.nlm.nih.gov/pmc/articles/PMC3275668/ (Accessed on 14 May 2019).
7. Wexler, P., Gilbert, S., Mohapatra, A., & Hakkinen, P., (2009). Information Resources in Toxicology (4th edn.). [eBook] San Diego: Elsevier Inc. Available at: http://file:///C:/Users/DEV/Desktop/P.J.%20Bert%20Hakkinen,%20Asish%20Mohapatra,%20Steven%20G.%20G.%20Gilbert,%20Philip%20Wexler%20-%20Information%20Resources%20in%20Toxicology,%20Fourth%20Edition-Academic%20Press%20(2009).pdf (Accessed on 14 May 2019).
8. Williams, P., (2012). Food Toxicity and Safety. [online] Pdfs.semanticscholar.org. Available at: https://pdfs.semanticscholar.org/5929/c425e7253093792dc9751fd9616c996507b7.pdf (Accessed on 14 May 2019).

Chapter 8

Current Advances and Future Challenges of Food Toxicology

CONTENTS

8.1. INTRODUCTION

The study of toxicology holds a true study of poisons, and it is a kind of chemical substance that entering in the body of human beings that can be more harmful and can cause adverse side effects. It has become modern science, and other sciences have been lacking unique methodologies or topics. Nowadays, there are a variety of foods, and these different foods have different toxins which may be referred to as the basic science of poisons. The challenge that human beings are facing is that they may be led to impaired health.

The chemicals have been hidden in the food, but all matters to the people are that the food should be delicious, and living organisms should like the food. So, the chemicals in the food have been added, but the people don't have the required information for each food product that there are more than thousands of chemicals that have been added in the food and they are also available in the market.

There are several advantages to using plastics for food packaging. Fluid and moldable, plastics can be made into sheets, shapes, and structures, offering considerable design flexibility. Because they are chemically resistant, plastics are inexpensive and lightweight with a wide range of physical and optical properties. Many plastics are heat sealable, easy to print, and can be integrated into production processes where the package is formed, filled, and sealed in the same production line. The major disadvantage of plastics is their variable permeability to light, gases, vapors, and low molecular weight molecules.

Some examples are iodized salt, folic acid added to flour, vitamin A added to oils/fats. The increasing occurrence of illnesses and diseases like diabetes and heart disease and anxiety about wellness has made it essential for experts to change the nutrient satisfaction of foods, for example, plummeting the calorie gratified of treated foods in numerous ways such as consuming false inducements.

The making of food has not been changed for a year because the chemicals are easily absorbed, which may provide the taste or change the colour of the food. But the food scientists use chemicals because it is the basic science of toxicology as it includes pharmacology, pathology, biochemistry, and to great measure chemistry.

Different types of food have been accepted by millions of people. But many foods contain toxins as a naturally occurring constituent or formed as a result of handling or processing.

Manufacturers are also playing a major role by setting limits on certain substances and developing mitigation procedures for process-induced toxins.

It has been observed that many toxins are present in commonly consumed foods, and certain toxins cannot be absorbed easily.

The protective approach which may be applied in certain cases is not considered as valued current and present chemicals and thus because chemistry classes will not be clear to clinical traits because of false accusations.

Testing of food is done by the food scientists as they must investigate it safely and efficiently followed by the health and safety rules. It is important to check that how many solutions are added and after doing the food test experiment, then they know how much they can use the more chemicals and solutions to it.

Every new product has been made with some chemicals including nanoparticles which improve organisms, cellular therapies, biologicals which are beyond basic requirements of nutritional value.

The food scientists believe that the risk should be less with the more consumption of food, and sometimes, the chemicals may create more demand for the foods. In the future, people will not cook with vegetables, fruit, or meat but with pure chemical compounds which should be responsible for the smell and taste of the food.

Many food industries have started to add a large number of flavours in the food which will change the reality of the food, and most people are aware of the idea that the food is naturally made up of chemical compounds.

Chemicals are everywhere in the world, which is considered as the building blocks. Food is not only consisting of chemicals, but it also includes plants, people, and animals. It is important to discuss the food varieties which is largely been consumed by the people and to know whether it has been harming the human body or not.

The survey is necessary to analyze the variety of toxicological properties which may affect the animals as well as the plants. The nutrients such as protein, fat, carbohydrates, and fiber are composed of chemical compounds. Toxicology occurs naturally in the food and contributes to the eating experience as well as a rounded diet.

Several food products like instant soup mixes and ready-to-cook items such as meals that are developed particularly cooking to the needs of working women. Additionally, the food industry has developed the strategy to add more nutrition at the time of making the packaged food products so that the consumers can purchase the food in a large amount of quantity.

Some chemicals in the food are not harmful to the human body, but they don't have proper nutritional value also. There are three types of biomarkers which are classified as biomarkers of susceptibility, biomarkers of effect, and biomarkers of effect. Selection of suitable biomarkers to measure the possible health-related outcomes and risk of experience to population subgroups and individuals. The characteristics and usefulness of pertinent technical considerations and analytical methods.

The food that the people purchased from the markets has some chemicals in them, but some chemicals have been added for future purposes, so that the food will last for longer as well as for improving production. There are many reasons why chemicals have been added to the food. Sometimes, it is necessary to add the chemicals in the food as the chemicals help the food not the change of colour in the future.

The people know the actual colour of the food, and they want the same food in the market. Sometimes, the colour of the food may change when they seem not so fresh, but chemicals help to keep the fruits clean, safe, and fresh for a longer time. By adding extra chemicals, there has been a risk to human health. It means that it should not affect the lives of humans. According to the survey, artificial colours have been added to the foods so that the food products look natural.

It has been observed that toxic chemicals may enter the food through packaging, and nowadays every product requires packaging as there are heavy metals in packaging that would collect in recycled materials to levels that presented serious health concerns. It will result in negative health effects, and children may be most at risk. The chemicals which have been added internally by the food scientists believed that these chemicals are safe. On the other hand, the chemicals that are potentially concerning are practically everywhere, even in dust, and it is impossible to avoid completely.

The chemicals outside the food product are completely different from the inside and outside chemicals are more dangerous than the inside chemicals. So, most of the food products should be washed from outside, so it will not harm human's health. The question has been raised that the food should consist of all nutritious value, but they get majorly get destroyed with the packaging.

For example, some of the most concerning are mixed into packaging, food wraps as well as plastic containers. The person's health is not being blamed for the chemicals that have been added to the food, but the person might have eaten something wrong, and the body may fail to digest which leads to food poisoning. If the food product contains the wrong chemicals, then it should be tested again and banned by the government in the future.

According to the recent studies, the smell, good taste and the most importantly the colour attract a greater number of people, and the chemicals do not certainly affect the human's health, but it decreases the nutritional value from the food. There have been thousands of chemicals that have been put into foods, and these chemicals have been increasing for the future. As a result, people will demand more variety if they like the taste, smell, and colour of the food. The studies state that healthy foods keep on fighting diseases with the increasing assault of harmful chemicals. There are major instruments in the food testing laboratories, and the machine can do 100 testings in a minute. Nobody can run from the food whether it has large number of chemicals which might affect the people's life because it has become the necessity of life.

8.2. TOXIC CHEMICALS THREATEN CURRENT AND FUTURE GENERATIONS

The toxic chemicals or substances endanger current as well as future generations. To secure them, people should alter the course by changing their chemical practices to a more sustainable model. The data present globally represents the increasing pressure on the environment because of the wastes and various other toxic chemicals (Figure 8.1).

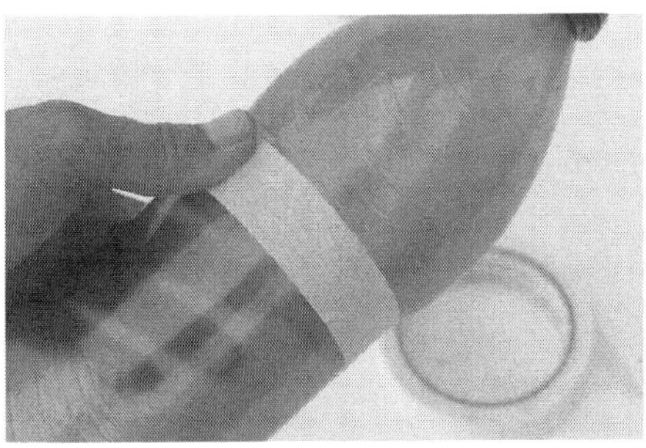

Figure 8.1. Chemicals in plastics.

Source: http://www.imagedoc.org/how-to-make-bangles-at-home-with-plastic-bottles/

The transfer of production of numerous chemicals to the transitions and developing nations has been complemented by a rise in the pesticide use, processes, and products having disease-causing chemicals- consisting of those that interrupt the process of reproduction, cause several birth defects, and remain in the bodies of human as well as environment causing harms.

Not so strong national legislation, sparse or even non-existent data and information regarding the health and environmental effects of the toxic chemicals, absence of funding and deprived human and technological resources in the developing economies make these nations susceptible to and disproportionally affected by the hazards of toxic chemicals.

Food scientists observe the quality of food and experiment by adding or removing chemicals because they know physical sciences, engineering, and biology so that they can study the arrangement of foods, and these changes occur at certain stages from produce through changes storage and processes. Food scientists work in the laboratory and check the quality of the food, and the foods get checked by them, and they must have the proper license.

Though developed nations empower their health and environmental legislation, transition, and developing, nations are still fighting with the issues that are not regarded as an issue in the developed nations anymore. A key example is the presence of lead in paint; it still constitutes a threat to children in developing economies (Figure 8.2).

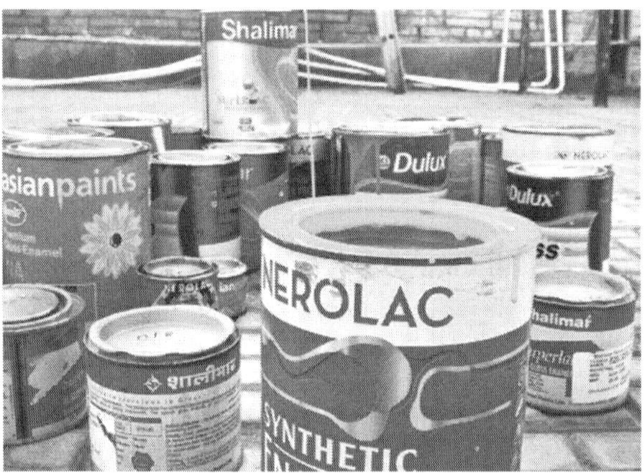

Figure 8.2. Presence of lead in paint.

Source: https://www.cseindia.org/lead-in-paints-521

Several individuals are still struggling with the accumulations of obsolete and expelled pesticides that pollute their food, water, and soil, damaging the health of humans as well as wildlife. They have been transformed into dumping grounds for novel hazardous pesticides that are previously banned in the developed nations but manufactured by their companies and marketed to the developing nations in a hostile way.

Children are born with dozens of hazardous chemicals in their bodies. Besides previously known toxic chemicals, huge numbers are introduced into the market per year. Most of them are not regulated by the current chemical conventions or by national legislation. Although, there is a lack of information regarding toxic chemicals and protective regulation.

Theoretically, they cause analogous harm to that from known toxic chemicals such as mercury or various other persistent organic pollutants (POPs). The disclosing chemicals that are utilized in the production process should be a universal standard to reduce the risks or chances of exposure that leads to suffering as well as a burden on the health system and economic development of countries.

An endemic burden of the disease and disability linked with the exposure to toxic chemicals is being witnessed by humans these days that eventually causes irreversible changes in the existing generations and will negatively impact the life of upcoming generations.

Several of these toxic chemicals harm the child along with the pregnant woman resulting in distressing lifelong and inter-generational consequences. Exposure to lead alone can cause harmful mental disabilities in almost 600,000 children annually, according to the World Health Organization (WHO). Subsistence gold miners, women, and their children breathe in vapors of mercury as they work to make a living.

Children living all around the world play with those toys that are made up of toxic plastics and endocrine-disrupting chemicals. In addition to that, some nations are still dependent on pesticides that can harm the brain of children and eventually lead to cancer.

Food scientists will evaluate the nutritional value so that it provides healthy food to the consumers. The food samples have been tested in the experimental labs for checking any chemicals or bacteria that have not been entered into the food and make sure that food manufacturing processes conform with government, processing, consumer, and industry standards. They understand the nature and the properties of food while dealing with the physicochemical aspects of food.

A great number of industries and the government must take a serious step to meet the Sustainable Development Goals by averting children from being exposed to toxic chemicals and pollution, together with substances whose risks are not well understood.

The initial steps beside this path consist of replacing the hazardous chemical components with safe substitutes in the processes and products and banning the goods comprising hazardous substances- including the ingredients present in household products such as paints and long-shelf-life food.

In some cases, it will be required to ban some chemicals completely, such as burning hazardous and unsegregated waste, comprising plastic and e-waste. Science, technology, and agricultural knowledge must not pose any health and environment-related threats, but should enhance the rural livelihoods, and enable equitable and sustainable development and socially, economically, and environmentally viable.

Chemical safety is inherent in many, if not all, of the sustainable development goals, but usually it is invisible and sidelined. Now, it is time to take action on chemical pollution so that the goals of sustainable development can be attained.

According to the studies, food chemistry is mainly involving in the physical, biological, and chemical makeup of food. It takes the applications for basic food preservation and food processing. The scientific disciplines in food technology are involved in engineering, chemistry, nutrition, and microbiology which have been applied for the nutrition, safety, availability, and wholesomeness of food that needs to be improved.

For sustainability, it is important to move to a circular economy, but recycling materials that include toxic chemicals only contaminate new products and sustains the exposure. There are data available that shows that the toxic chemicals obtained from the e-waste have been recycled into toys even in the developed nations.

The recycling materials that comprise toxic chemicals or compounds, including those which are already debarred by the international treaties, destroy the supply chain as well as the circular economy and weakens the significance of recycling.

Healthy and nutritious food helps people to fight the harmful diseases that people are faced with the rising assault of harmful and hazardous chemicals in human bodies. Two new studies recently found fluorinated chemicals that can percolate into the food during the packaging process, take-out packages, and French fries boxes, and microwave popcorn bags.

These studies eventually add to a developing body of research finding injurious chemicals hidden in our food supply. These chemicals consist of hormone-disrupting phthalates and cancer-causing perfluorinated chemicals. Even toxic flame retardants can end up in food.

Nutrients should be well conserved, which contains some essential minerals and vitamins. The food Scientists may add more nutrition to the food products and toxic principles and chemicals will not be added; otherwise, it will increase the risk of disease with the bad food.

Some of these hazardous chemicals get into the food as they are deliberately used in the packaging of food or are present in the equipment used for food processing. Some may also enter the supply of food as they are present in the soil, air, and water used to grow the food.

These days, food security is a major concern of people. People must not have to worry regarding the offensive chemicals gratuitously contaminating the food and making people sick. That is why; toxic-free future is increasing the issue focus to struggling for toxic-free food! Companies who sell food have accountability to keep unwanted harmful chemicals out of their products. The policymakers should confine the existence of toxic chemicals in food.

8.3. ADVANCES IN THE DEVELOPMENT OF ALTERNATIVES TO WHOLE ANIMAL (VERTEBRATE) TESTING

As animal examination has now become a kind of emotional issue, it is crucial to identify the increasing effect of in vitro toxicology on the exercise of toxicology. However, this field is generally known as "alternative," and the experimental models have been used to the 3Rs of Russel and Burch.

- To REPLACE the models of animals;
- To REDUCE the number of animals utilized;
- To REFINE the test methods to decrease the stress as well as the suffering of animals.

In the context of toxicology, "alternatives to whole animal or vertebrate experimentation" usually refers to in vitro tests for the latent toxicity that substitutes for or replaces in vivo (whole animal) studies. "In vitro" exactly means "in glass" and is understood to mean "outside of the body" or "in a test tube."

The alternative tests comprise short-term tests by utilizing isolated cells, tissues, and organs. The studies including epidemiology, mathematical modeling, or the use of human volunteers; short-term tests for genetic toxicity are excluded.

Practically, alternative test methods are used to support the process of planning as well as interpretation of the overall studies of animal toxicity, and yet are not used as alternatives for the toxicity studies using animals. For instance, an alternate test can be used:

- To regulate the virtual biological strength of a chain of toxicants at the cellular level.
- To choose the animal model to conduct an in vivo test by relating the metabolic properties of a toxicant at the cellular level in numerous species.
- To recognize mechanism(s) of toxicity by outlining the relationship between exposure to a toxicant and growth of several toxicological endpoints at the cellular, subcellular, and molecular levels of the organization.

Current advances that have been made in in-vitro studies with isolated cells or tissues or organs have focused the scientific community towards developing, authorizing, and assessing substitute test systems. The analytical value of an identical test must be evaluated utilizing a sequence of validation studies.

Although, the technology used in packaging the products that will help in balancing the food protection without getting into trouble. To transfer the food, it includes energy and material costs, heightened environmental and social awareness, and strict laws on the removal of community solid waste and pollutants or chemicals.

Validation can determine that using an in vitro test is similar to the use of a traditional in vivo test or that the in vivo test forecasts the human activity accurately. Expecting a regular increase in the development as well as the use of alternative in vitro test systems, various agencies and communities boost the development of approaches that can provide relevant information to the evaluation of human risks.

8.3.1. Developing Alternative Tests

There are various reasons to enforce the development of alternate in vitro tests. Some of them are listed below:

- ***Economy and Efficiency***: In vitro tests may provide the information related to toxicity once established, in a time-saving as well as cost-effective manner. The information produced from in vitro test systems can further be utilized to increase the efficacy of whole-animal studies and reduce the number of animals used in the testing methods of toxicity. The simplicity, as well as space-saving features of in vitro methods, is considered as effective advantages.
- ***Information about Human Risk***: Human cells that are obtained ethically and established in vitro successfully, may eventually provide relevant information regarding a specific toxicant related to human risk and diseases. For instance, the metabolism or mechanism of action of a toxicant present in a human cell can provide the base for selecting an appropriate animal model for long-term toxicity studies (Figure 8.3).

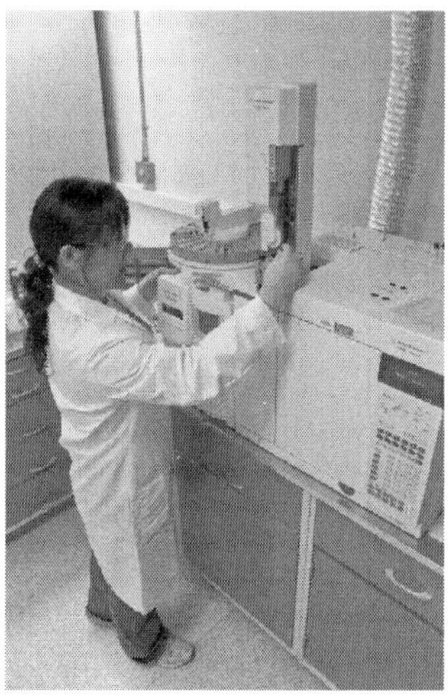

Figure 8.3. Testing food in the laboratory.

Source: https://www.flickr.com/photos/fdaphotos/6008498003'

8.3.2. Possible Applications of Alternative Tests

The isolated cells, tissues, and organs can easily be prepared and sustained in culture by using those methods that protect the properties or characteristics of the same cells, tissues, or organs in vivo. Using these kinds of in vitro systems will allow data to be produced under controlled experimental conditions and in the absence of various complicating factors specific to experiments with whole animals.

For instance, the utilization of cell culture systems will make able the metabolism of a toxicant that takes place in one type of cell be separately studied from a toxic endpoint that takes place in a different type of cell.

Various toxic endpoints may provide themselves to quantification in an in-vitro test system. The relevant and appropriate endpoints could be recognized by equating the action of toxicants at molecular, subcellular, and cellular sites with the toxic effects found in the target tissue or organ in vivo. The investigation of a broad range of in vitro cellular events may provide relevant information regarding the in vivo development of a toxic response as a function of toxicant concentration as well as time.

As in vitro techniques have the strength to produce reproducible measurements; theoretically, they lend themselves to normalization. Although, inferring data acquired from a normalized in vitro toxicity test with a practical level of confidence can only take place after potential difficult factors like the interactions between the non-cellular components and the test agent of the test system have been recognized or eliminated.

The validation process seems to be crucial for the complete acceptance of the alternative tests where the relevance, as well as reliability of procedures, is established for definite purposes. A huge number of components seem crucial for overall coordination of the process of validation, including the scientific agreement on the explanation of a validated test, reference chemicals with general availability and distinct toxicity, a central source for test performance data and protocols, a recognized network of laboratories with the abilities of method validation, as well as scientific understanding of the basis of the toxicological process involved.

A competent and impartial group of scientists from different regulatory agencies and the research communities could facilitate the execution of the validation process.

Food chemistry can delay product fall as well as hold the positive effects of dispensation, increase or maintain the safety and quality of food, and extend shelf-life. As a result, packaging protects every food product from three major concepts of outside impacts such as chemical, physical, and biological.

The chemical or bacteria generally enter in the open food product and most people do not prefer open food products and environmental influences on the food products like expose of gases mainly oxygen gas and moisture like gain or loss or light like infrared, visible, and ultraviolet (UV). The food industry uses different food techniques like packing the products in a very different way. It means every different food product should have a different kind of packaging.

8.3.3. Limitations of Alternative Tests

There are a huge number of limitations of in vitro tests, and these are already known. For example:

In vitro test systems are not present for all tissues as well as organs. Furthermore, the normal systemic procedure of absorption, permeation, supply, and emission are not present in vitro test systems. In vitro systems do not have the complex, cooperative effects of the immune, endocrine systems, blood, nervous system, and various other integrated elements of the whole animal.

Hence, in vitro tests cannot be utilized in studying the complex nature of systemic activity. The standardization of modern methods is expensive as well as time-consuming; acceptance of in vitro tests as a substitute for traditional toxicity testing methods in whole animals is assumed to be slow. Though numerous schemes have been anticipated to accelerate these processes. At present, no alternative in vitro test can replace an in vivo study of toxicity.

8.3.4. Current Use of In Vitro Tests

A great number of divers in vitro tests have been recently developed. These tests will be enhanced in quality over time by the introduction of modern technological advances and scientific information in the field of in vitro toxicology and its related fields like biotechnology and molecular biology.

The use and development of in vitro test systems are mainly encouraged for planning as well as interpreting the outcomes obtained from whole animal toxicity studies. Crucial advancements have been recently made in the development of in vitro substitutes for visual safety testing. Several other in vitro systems have also been proposed which calculate a wide range of endpoints, and at present in different stages of the validation.

The agencies or communities currently working in the field of toxicology are a part of interagency regulatory groups that are assessing or evaluating the proposed alternative test methods. The in vitro approaches to toxicity testing can eventually provide useful data when it is combined with any other information regarding the toxicity of food as well as the colour additives that are used in food.

The outcomes of an in vitro test can be utilized to optimize the structure of traditional toxicity tests for a specific test substance by aiding to regulate the levels of dose and by aiding to decide which species are the signature model for humans.

Such kind of improvements in the structure of toxicity tests of whole animals may decrease the number of test animals needed to produce relevant information regarding the safety of the food additives used in food. In vitro tests can also help in clarifying the nature of the interaction between the organism and test substance at the cellular, subcellular, and molecular levels.

Sometimes, the structure of the food products is not similar, and the packing of the food products also looks different. Metals and glass offer an almost complete barrier to many environmental agents and chemicals. On the other hand, but few packages are absolutely or purely metal or glass as the end devices are added to ease both exhausting and filling.

Hence, once the crucial target organ or the organ system has been recognized in the studies of the whole animal, in vitro tests can easily concentrate on the mechanism of action of the test substance at the specific target site.

Significant information from these studies can help the agencies in taking decisions regarding the safety of proposed colour additives added in food by analyzing the responses observed in the animal and human cells, and also by simplifying extrapolation to low-dose from high-dose responses.

Currently, in assessing a request for using a food additive, the agencies consider in vitro tests to be quite significant and useful in recognizing the mechanism of action of the test substance and to give information related to indirect effects observed in vitro that may not be seen in vivo studies.

8.4. TOXIC CHEMICALS IN OUR FOOD SYSTEM

Chemicals are nowadays used in every single step of the food production process, whether it is the step of production, harvesting, processing, packing, transporting, marketing, and consumption. This can be quite dangerous for the health of humans. Some of these hazardous chemicals sustain in the food and environment for decades.

It is not allowed to add extra chemicals to the food, and intentional interfering with the food and medicinal products is not allowed; thus, the packaging in the products is necessary and useful. Especially pharmaceutical products require special packaging features that will help in reducing the threat of adulteration and tampering.

But in case, any package can have tamper-evident and can be breached features that cannot easily be exchanged. The features of temper evident are breakaway closures, special printing, banding, and special membranes on composite cans or bottle liners such as text or graphics that forever change from time to time.

For example, the tamper-evident feature that will no longer give extra packaging materials is a heat seal which has been seen on the medical packaging, which will result in chemically expressed to change shade when it gets unlocked.

Preservatives are mainly added to various processed food products, including cereals, meat, and bread. Recent studies have found that additives are the major source of nausea, headache, breathing difficulties, weakness, etc. Currently conducted research has revealed that they might damage the nerve cells of human beings. They could have long-term effects on human health as synthetic additives are a new invention.

Few of the fishes comprise toxic chemicals known as polychlorinated biphenyls (PCBs). They have been debarred earlier but remain in the environment and end up in the food system or heavy metals such as mercury. PCBs can easily destruct the developing brains of children and have been associated with various behavioural disorders. Heavy metals such as mercury may decrease the IQ level and cause hearing or visual impairment.

Food packaged in plastics may have phthalates or various other hazardous chemicals. As the chemicals can leak from the packaging into the food itself, they can cause harmful diseases. Research has connected phthalates to behavioural disorders. Glass containers give various benefits in making the food safe in terms of food packaging applications because it is chemically and unscented with almost every food product. The glass containers have been designed in such a way that has become resistant to vapors and gases. As a result, it will make the product fresh for a longer period without harming the flavour or taste.

8.4.1. Avoid Toxic Foods in Future

The food toxicants cannot be avoided entirely in the food. Several steps can be taken to decrease our current as well as future exposure. These steps may include- choosing organic and sustainable options. The intake of pesticides can be reduced by avoiding the consumption of fruits and vegetables that are contaminated.

Help institutions like hospitals and schools in buying safe and sustainable food. With their huge potential of purchasing, these institutions can make a crucial impact on the health of people and eventually, the community.

From students and teachers in the school to the patients, visitors, and staff in the hospital, a great number of people spend money and consume different food products in these institutions every day. Boost these institutions to buy those food products that are sustainable and harmless.

Demand local and national food, farm, and chemical policy changes. People are required to make a good national investment in enforcing an efficient agricultural, environmental, and food policy that supports the sustainable or viable practices of production on farms. Policy change is very much needed to renovate the current system. Individuals can support viable agricultural policies by just contacting their legislators.

8.5. AVOID TOXIC CHEMICALS IN FUTURE

- ***Limit Canned Food and Plastic Containers*:** Lead-free ceramic, glass, and stainless steel are known as great substitutes to store food in plastic containers. One of the major exposures to the toxic chemical BPA is the canned food. A recent study conducted by the Breast Cancer Fund as well as the Silent Spring Institute observed that families can easily decrease their levels of BPA by 60% in three days by evading food packaging with BPA (Figure 8.4).

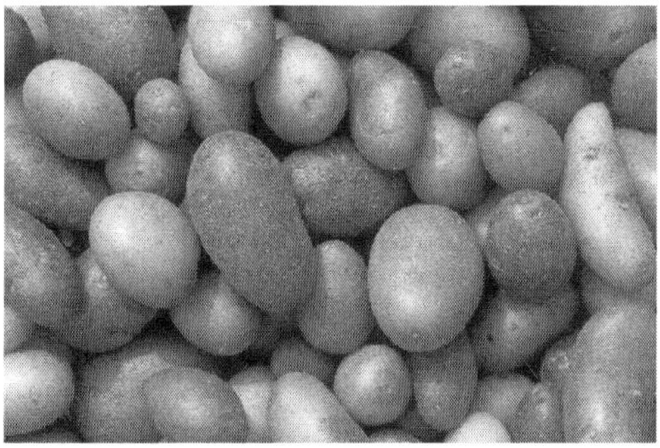

Figure 8.4. Avoid toxic foods.

Source: https://en.wikipedia.org/wiki/Potato

- ***Avoid Non-Stick Pans***: They can appear useful or suitable, but be cautious of the non-stick pans. Most of the non-stick cookware is made up of PFOA (perfluorooctanoic acid), which is a toxic chemical associated with cancer and various other severe health-related issues. Instead, go for stainless steel, enameled, or cast iron pots and cans.
- ***Popcorn the Old Fashioned Way:*** The microwave popcorn bags are lined with the hazardous PFOA. This carcinogen eventually shows up in the pizza boxes and French fry cups. People should fry the popcorn on the stove or use a brown paper bag while microwaving.
- ***Filter Your Drinking Water***: Eliminate hazardous contaminants such as lead and arsenic from the drinking water by the process of filtration with a water pitcher or a faucet unit. Avoid purchasing plastic water bottles, instead of the plastic bottles fill up a bottle made up of stainless steel.
- ***Buy Organic When Possible***: Before heading to the grocery store, people should check out the list of dirty dozen. Organic doesn't always have to be more expensive as compared to pesticide-laden food. Various farmers' markets, as well as communities, supported agriculture programs, have healthy produce, which is cost-competitive.
- ***Avoid food dyes***: Food items present in the market include food dyes, 90% of which are mainly obtained from petroleum. Recent studies show that dyes are directly related to hyperactivity and several other disturbing behaviours in humans.

- ***Tell Congress to Fix Our Broken Laws***: Enough with this nonsense! Consumers should not have to tackle the load of avoiding or neglecting toxic chemicals.

8.6. STEPS TO AVOID TOXIC CHEMICALS IN DAY-TO-DAY LIFE

Step 1: Making your products of cleaning

It is easy, cheap, and fun to make the cleaners having no toxicity, from effective and safe ingredients such as baking soda and vinegar. This will decrease the risk of asthma, cancer, and hormone disruption.

Step 2: Avoid Fragrance

Shop for laundry detergents, cleaners, personal care products characterized as "fragrance-free." People should keep in mind that "Unscented" does not always mean fragrance-free! People should not use any room fresheners.

Fragrance can be composed of a variety of chemicals that companies are allowed to keep secret from the customers. The common chemical fragrance comprises synthetic musks that are associated with an increased risk of breast cancer and phthalates that are associated with reproductive and developmental harm.

Step 3: Give Your Personal Care Products a Makeover

People should always read the label of products to avoid chemicals such as oxybenzone, sodium laureth sulphate, and parabens. The use of such products should be very less. The products of personal care include a broad range of chemicals; some of them are known to be of great concern while many are deprived of research to prove safety. These products are applied to the skin and hence get absorbed easily into the body.

Step 4: Go "BPA-Free."

Discard the channel foods whenever possible and go for fresh or frozen vegetables and fruits. People should opt for those products that are packaged in a glass or lined cardboard as an alternative to cans.

Bisphenol-A (BPA) is usually found in can liners and plastic products. Exposure to BPA is associated with a host of hormone-related health impacts like increased risk of infertility, cancer, diabetes, and obesity.

Step 5: Quit the Quats

People should not use disinfectant products and avoid antibacterial soaps, sanitizers, and various cleaning products that include quaternary ammonium compounds (quats). The front label should always be checked to avoid the products which comprise ingredients that are hazardous to the human body. This will lead to the promotion of antibacterial-resistant bacteria ("super-bugs").

Step 6: Wherever Possible Choose Alternatives to Plastics

To store the food, use ceramic bowls or glass jars. People must keep in mind that plastics are not meant for microwave things. Plastics should be washed only by hands, not in the dishwater. Avoid using plastics having recycled symbols #3 for PVC, #6 for polystyrene, and #7 for others which have a major potential to percolate toxins and they are difficult to recycle.

Magnesium and manganese are frequently added to aluminium to improve its strength properties. Unlike many metals, aluminium is extremely unaffected to most procedures and methods of weathering and rust; its natural covering of aluminium oxide delivers a highly real fence to the belongings and properties of moisture, air, chemical attack, and temperature.

The products of plastic can have various toxic additives like heavy metals, phthalates, and several other compounds that leach out over time. Polyvinyl chloride (PVC) is also known as poison plastic, and it is mainly found in plastic products from toys to cookware to shower curtains.

Step 7: Keep Harmful Chemicals Out of the House

Take off shoes before entering the house to avoid tracking in oils as well as chemicals from the street outside. People can use a doormat to latch dirt at the door only. Houses should be regularly cleaned with HEPA filter vacuum as dust carries hazardous chemicals that shed off of electronics, furniture, and numerous other household products.

Step 8: Turn Down the Heat on Non-Stick Cookware

While using non-stick or Teflon cookware, keep the stove at medium heat. Go for stainless steel or cast iron pans for cooking purposes. Teflon produces PFOA when heated to 450 degrees. PFOA is related to developmental harm as well as cancer.

Step 9: Ditch the Air Fresheners

Eradicate odour: Recognize the smell and prevent it.

Open the window: Ventilating the home with outdoor air has been observed to decrease the symptoms that are linked with infections, allergies, and asthma. People should set out a bouquet of fresh flowers to add a floral scent to the home. Several of the air fresheners that are regularly used in our homes add redundant chemicals, including those also that may degrade our homes.

Step 10: Join Women's Voices for the Earth!

People should implement their potential to assure a safe and healthy future. Donate to the efforts of reducing the toxic or hazardous chemicals that affect the health of women.

8.7. CONCLUSION

It is important to have a toxic-free future. Plastics play a major role in making the food affected and generate new chemicals in the food because plastics have been considered cheap, convenient, and ubiquitous as they create permanent pollution and they leach chemicals that contaminate the drink and the food. The government has also warned consumers to reduce the use of plastics because of several reasons.

The students may have chosen the subjects like Biology, physics, and chemistry, or some other stream-like mathematics. Alternative courses are biotechnology, microbiology, biochemistry, organic chemistry, chemical/ process engineering, nutrition, and pharmaceutical sciences, which have also been associated with Food Science or Food Engineering.

Food science and technology both are vast topics to be plotted as an essay. Food science can be included in foods. It may include the chemical composition of the food; storage and its effects are explained. It is the study of the complete physical, chemical, and biological effects of food.

The government has also banned plastics to keep the remaining food safe for the future as it has largely impacted the food, and due to plastics, many people have suffered from the disease. These biomarkers are, among others, tools to evaluate the risk and possible health-related outcomes to individuals and population subgroups. Because of their increasing availability and sensitivity, biomarkers are increasingly being used to explore the links between exposure and effect to establish causality.

The contrast between individual variability and common characteristics becomes important to understand how behavioural phenotypes, constructed as an environmentally driven diet physiological adaptation, influence susceptibility to food toxicants.

People generally store the food in plastics, which is not good. Even the shopkeepers are not allowed to give the food products in the plastics which usually contain chemical additives which are not being evaluated for safety. Steel is the best option for keeping the food safe as it is better than plastics. It is important to discuss plastics because plastics end up in the garbage, accumulating in oceans, polluting on especially harmful land.

Packaging food in plastics will bring chemicals that decrease the quality and safety of food. Many times, the food which has been tested in the laboratory is safer and clean as was suggested by the various food organizations. But when it comes to the market, the food doesn't remain fresh, clean, and healthy because various chemicals will exist in the food due to external influences like pollution or plastics.

The food is not been directly or openly sold to the consumers as every food needs packaging. It has been observed that external chemicals that have been existed in food products will not get blamed by various food associations or companies. But they use different packaging for different products to save the products from chemicals. It has been largely observed that the food from outside looks unclean, which means that the food has been destroyed, but from inside, the food is fresher and healthier because the chemicals have affected the food from outside. On the other hand, the food from the outside looks good but deep inside it has affected by chemicals, and the chemical has failed to keep the food safe for a longer period.

Biological protection gives safety to the food and stops chemicals to enter the food, including spoiling and pathogens agents. Many food products justify that they are artificial flavoured, and it has been mentioned in the food label that it is called a flavoured product. The target of the food organization and associations is to add the chemicals in each food product to sell more food items, and that is why chemistry has helped the modern world in various ways.

Food that has been damaged, crushed, or expired is a different thing, but chemicals have become important for the food as they have multiple functions in the food. It is not like that the food which has been made from the farming are direct eaten by the consumers but it went for testing, packaging, and at that time the food scientists check the level of the food and they use the chemicals for keeping the food safety in the future. Most of the processed foods that are available in the market have a long life varying between a few months to even a few years. It has become possible because the right chemicals have existed in such foods. Chemicals also perform some other functions like improving the physical appearance of the food for the future, and various chemicals will help the producers boost the appeal and make them more attractive to consumers. The chemicals have been used for cosmetic purposes.

Putting chemicals in the food has been increasing, and there has been a large number of demands for chemical food products as they are giving the taste, great colour as well as nutritional value to foods. The goal of every food organization is to add colours, artificial flavours, preservatives, supplements, artificial sweeteners, stabilizing agents, and trans-fat, and these chemicals are giving profit to the various food industries. The food industries have replaced old and natural food products with artificial product. For example, sugar now has been coming as artificial sweetener, and it has been changing due to chemistry.

The chemistry is coming up with alternatives because the natural food gets expired or destroyed very early and foods get spoiled in a shorter time, and there has been a growth of microorganisms as well as microbes. So, the chemicals have introduced the alternative food, and the chemical food is controlled easily, which has resulted in increasing the Shelf life of the food. It has been noticed that the packaged foods have a longer life, which can consume weeks and months. The chemicals as well the packaging has kept the food safer for the future, but large quantities of chemicals may have ill effects on human health.

Food chemicals are the application of food science to the selection, preservation, processing, packaging, distribution, and use of safe food technology. Food technology is a branch of food science that deals with the production processes that make foods. Early scientific research into food technology concentrated on food preservation. Food Science and technology is the branch that completely describes the preservation, processing, and packaging of food.

There are various reasons for processing food items. Nowadays, when the grains get dried after harvesting, then it will result in a rising shelf life. Before that, foods were handled mainly to improve palatability, digestibility, and to make sure there is a continuous supply of food items. In Asian countries, the pickles, papads, and murabbas have been used so much by the people who are called the preserved products that have been made from grains and fruits or vegetables.

There has been a great demand for packaged food products that have been fresher, more natural, healthier, and safe foods and it has more consumed by a large number of people, and package food allows suitable shelf life. Food science has also improved the transportation system, and transportation is the key source in food science. The food and dairy industry is mostly depending on the timely and smooth supply of food products.

Consumers know what to purchase, and they want a good quality of foods when they went to the market as they search for better quality food and the consumers like some attractive packing in the food. Before purchasing the package food products, they look for the following nutrition's for that product along with the good taste if the consumer is purchasing for the first time. There are some foods that can easily be packed, store, and transport.

The food product should have Convenience features, which include product visibility, resealability, handling, ease of access, and disposal that largely impact package innovation. As a result, packaging plays a major role in diminishing the effort required to serve and prepare foods. Microwavable packaging, oven-safe trays, and biol-in bags allow consumers to cook and eat the entire meal with almost no preparation.

Package construction and package design will play an important role in defining the shelf life of a food product. Firstly, the sample of the foods is taken into the laboratory, and it gets tested and the food will be safe and clean then there should be a right selection of packaging materials so that the technologies will also help in maintaining the freshness and product quality during storage and distribution.

Nowadays, people look for everything, and they especially observe food products because they are often combining several resources and materials to expose each material's aesthetic or functional properties. According to the research, everybody is used to see some improvement in food packaging. Even the caps of the bottles get changed, and every time people see a new packet but with the same food.

REFERENCES

1. Advances in the Development of Alternatives to Whole Animal (Vertebrate) Testing, (n.d.). [eBook] p. 4. Available at: https://www.fda.gov/downloads/Food/GuidanceRegulation/GuidanceDocumentsRegulatoryInformation/IngredientsAdditivesGRASPackaging/UCM078780.pdf (Accessed on 14 May 2019).
2. Dahl, L., (2012). Tips to Avoid Toxic Chemicals in Food. [online] Saferchemicals.org. Available at: https://saferchemicals.org/2012/12/03/tips-to-avoid-toxic-chemicals-in-food/ (Accessed on 14 May 2019).
3. HEJ Support, (n.d.). New Article: Toxic Chemicals Threaten Current and Future Generations – HEJ Support. [online] Available at: https://hej-support.org/toxic-chemicals-threaten-current-future-generations-protect-must-change-course-shifting-chemical-practices-sustainable-model/ (Accessed on 14 May 2019).
4. Sachan, A., & Hendrich, S., (2019). Food Toxicology: Current Advances and Future Challenges. [eBook] p. 4.
5. Toxic Chemicals in Our Food System, (n.d.). [eBook] p. 4. Available at: https://www.psr.org/wp-content/uploads/2018/05/toxic-chemicals-in-our-food-system.pdf (Accessed on 14 May 2019).
6. Women's voices for the earth, (n.d.). 10 Steps to Avoid Toxic Chemicals. [online] Available at: https://www.womensvoices.org/avoid-toxic-chemicals/ten-ways-to-avoid-toxic-chemicals/ (Accessed on 14 May 2019).

INDEX

F

G

H

I